HEALING ME NOW

MARK FLORY

HEALING ME NOW

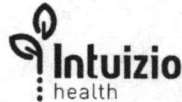

For Shannyn:
To my soulmate and the person who inspired me to look at myself and become healthy again. Your hard work, persistence, discipline, and drive to live a healthy lifestyle, have truly changed my life.
I will forever love you!

CONTENTS

Dedication
iii

— Table of Contents
1

1 — Healing Me Now
10

2 — The Resistance Begins
24

3 — Pushing The Limit
34

4 — The Pain of Progress
43

5 — The Breaking Point
52

6 — The Transformation Begins
61

7 — The Discipline Gap
69

8 – Breaking the Plateau
78

9 – Becoming the Man He Was Meant to Be
86

10 – The Turning Point
94

11 – Building the Future
102

12 – Leading the Way
110

13 – A New Standard
118

14 – The Lifestyle Shift
127

15 – The Healthy Mindset
134

16 – Final Thoughts
142

About the Author
146

TABLE OF CONTENTS

Introduction
Healing Me Now
Chapter 1: The Wake-Up Call
The Moment of Truth
A Conversation That Changes Everything
Facing the Hard Truth
The First Step is the Hardest
The Truth About Food

Chapter 2: The Resistance Begins
The First Temptation
Old Habits Die Hard
The Happy Hour Test
The Wings Showdown
Breaking the Cycle

Chapter 3: Pushing the Limits
The Wake-Up Call—Round Two
The Test of Endurance
Fighting Through the Pain
The Aftermath
Welcome to the Gym

Chapter 4: The Pain of Progress
Leg Day Hell
When Every Step Hurts
The Morning After
Pushing Through the Soreness
Strength Over Struggle

Chapter 5: The Breaking Point
When Doubt Creeps In
A Crossroads
The Hardest Morning Yet
Pushing Past the Wall
The Moment of Truth

Chapter 6: The Transformation Begins
Small Wins, Big Changes
When the Mirror Shows Progress
A New Routine
The First Real Test
The Food Battle

Chapter 7: The Discipline Gap
When Willpower is Tested
The Mental Game
Owning the Choice
When No One's Watching
The Late-Night Craving

Chapter 8: Breaking the Plateau
The Comfort Trap
The Next Level
The Sprint That Changed Everything

The Final Sprint
The Shift in Mindset

Chapter 9: Becoming the Man He Was Meant to Be
A New Standard
The Strength Test
The Mental Shift
The Unexpected Challenge
Commitment Over Convenience

Chapter 10: The Turning Point
The Moment It Clicked
Leading by Example
The Ripple Effect
Owning the New Identity
No More Limits

Chapter 11: Building the Future
The Next Step
Strength Beyond the Gym
The Shift No One Expected
The First Recruit
The Responsibility of Growth

Chapter 12: Leading the Way
Setting the Standard
The Test of Commitment
No More Halfway
Pushing Through the Wall
The Breakthrough

Chapter 13: A New Standard
The Shift That Sticks
The Challenge Outside the Gym
Balance Without Compromise
The Real Strength Test
Showing Up Where It Matters

Chapter 14: The Lifestyle Shift
The Moment It Became Normal
The Proof in the Mirror
The Unexpected Validation
The Final Piece of the Puzzle
A Life Fully Lived

Chapter 15: The Healing Mindset
The Strength in Simplicity
Becoming an Example
The Legacy of Discipline
The Journey Never Ends

Final Thoughts
There Is No One-Size-Fits-All Approach
Start Where You Are
My Journey Continues, Too
You Are Not Alone

INTRODUCTION

The Journey to Healing Starts Now

What if I told you that the biggest obstacle standing between you and the healthiest version of yourself isn't your age, genetics, or even your past choices—but your mindset?

For years, I believed that my body would always take care of itself. As a professional athlete, I never had to think about my workouts or my nutrition—performance was my focus, and the physical benefits came naturally. But life has a way of humbling us. Injuries forced me to stop playing, and as the years went on, I watched my body change in ways I never expected. The weight crept on. My joints ached. My energy dipped. Worst of all, my mind—once sharp and focused—felt sluggish, trapped in a cycle of frustration and self-doubt.

Then, one day, I hit my breaking point. A severe back injury left me unable to move for days. The pain wasn't just physical—it was a wake-up call. If I didn't take control of my health, my future would be one of limitations, medications, and regret. That wasn't an option. Not for me. And if you're reading this, I'm willing to bet that deep down, you feel the same way.

You're here because you know something needs to change. You're tired of the endless cycle of quick fixes, diets that don't stick, and workouts that leave you feeling more defeated than empowered. You want a real transformation—a stronger body, a sharper mind, and a life filled with purpose. But how do you get there?

That's where this journey begins.

The Trap of Instant Gratification

If there's one thing I've learned through my own struggles, it's this: most people fail at health and wellness because they're trapped in a cycle of **instant gratification**. We live in a world of quick results—fast food, overnight shipping, and instant downloads. So when we don't see immediate changes in our health, we get discouraged and quit. Sound familiar?

The truth is, real health isn't a destination—it's a journey. And like any worthwhile journey, it takes **discipline, consistency, and the right mindset** to stay the course. That's why this book isn't just about what to eat or how to exercise. Those things matter, but without the right mental foundation, no diet or workout plan will ever stick.

This book is about something much deeper. It's about **breaking free from the patterns that have**

held you back for years and finally stepping into the healthiest, strongest version of yourself.

A Different Approach to Health

Most health books focus on mechanics: eat this, lift that, stretch like this. And while those details are important, they miss a crucial piece of the puzzle—**your mindset**. If you don't change how you think about health, you'll keep repeating the same cycles over and over again.

That's why this book is different.

Instead of chasing the next "perfect" workout or diet plan, we'll start with the foundation—the way you think about your health and your body. Because when you shift your mindset, everything else starts to fall into place naturally. You'll begin to make better choices, not because you "have to," but because you **want to**. You'll stop seeing health as a chore and start embracing it as a lifelong journey.

This book is about **reprogramming your mind** so that healthy living becomes second nature. And once that happens? You'll be unstoppable.

The 4 Pillars of Healing

As you progress through this book and beyond, you'll be introduced to the **4 Pillars of Healing**—the core elements that will support your transformation:

Nutrition – Fueling your body with the right foods, not just for weight loss, but for long-term vitality.
Physical Activity – Moving in ways that strengthen and heal your body, regardless of your starting point.
Sleep – The foundation of recovery, energy, and mental clarity.
Self-Improvement – Cultivating a resilient mindset that keeps you motivated and inspired.

This book sets the foundation for these pillars. It's the starting point for your transformation, helping you develop the mental and emotional strength needed to follow through on any health plan—whether it's mine or someone else's.

Your Journey Starts Now

This isn't a quick-fix program. It's not about chasing an ideal body or fitting into a certain size. It's about something far more important—**creating a lifestyle that allows you to thrive** for years to come.
You might have tried and failed before. That's okay. This time will be different. Because this time, you won't just be changing your habits—you'll be

changing your entire approach to health. And when you do that, the results will last a lifetime.

So take a deep breath. Let go of the doubts and the past failures. You are here, right now, for a reason. This is your chance to rewrite your story—to reclaim your strength, your energy, and your purpose.

Are you ready? Then turn the page. Your journey to healing starts now.

HEALING ME NOW

Chapter 1: The Wake-Up Call

The Moment of Truth

David Carter sat at the edge of his bed, his breath shallow, heart pounding against his ribs like a warning drum. His fingers gripped the crumpled paper in his lap—the results from his latest medical check-up. High cholesterol, elevated blood pressure, pre-diabetic. Words he never thought he'd have to worry about, not at 46, not after a life spent in his prime as an athlete.

But here he was. He was overweight, sluggish, and battling a dull ache in his lower back that had become as constant as the morning sun. His once chiseled jawline had softened, his muscles had surrendered to time, and his energy levels felt like a drained battery struggling to recharge.

His doctor's voice echoed in his mind: *"David, you need to make serious changes, or the next warning sign might not be something you can overcome."*

It wasn't a casual suggestion. It was a line drawn in the sand, a moment that demanded a choice—stay on the path leading to an inevitable decline, or fight his way back.

His eyes drifted to the mirror across the room. He barely recognized the man staring back. His wife, Lisa, had always been gentle about his health, urging him to take better care of himself without pushing too hard. But last night, her concern had turned into something sharper.

"David, I'm scared. You're not yourself anymore. I miss the man who had the energy to take on the world."

He had brushed her off, muttering something about work stress and aging. But deep down, he knew the truth. He had let himself go.

A gust of wind rattled the bedroom window, and for the first time in years, he felt a chill that had nothing to do with the weather. It was the weight of reality pressing down on him.

He stood up, the soreness in his knees reminding him of the years of neglect. His mind raced. Where would he even start? He knew the drill—exercise, nutrition, better sleep—but knowing and doing were two different things.

Then his phone buzzed.

A message from an old friend.

"Dave, you've been on my mind lately. Let's catch up."

David frowned. "Whatever", he mumbled under his breath. He hadn't heard from Jake in years and now he wants to catch up.

And then, as if fate had pulled a string, he remembered—Jake had gone through a transformation himself a few years back. He too, was struggling with his own health crisis, and turned his life around in ways David had always admired from a distance.

A spark ignited in David's chest. Maybe this was the sign he needed.

He inhaled deeply and typed back: **"Hey, Jake great to hear from you. Lisa and I were just talking and I think I could use your help."**

Just as he hit send, a wave of apprehension rolled over him.

What if it was too late?

What if he couldn't change?

But somewhere, beneath the doubt, another voice whispered:

What if you can?

A Conversation That Changes Everything

David's phone remained in his hand long after he sent the message. He stared at the screen, his nerves tightening with each passing second. Would Jake even respond? It had been nearly a decade since they last spoke, and the silence stretched, pressing down on him like a weight.

His mind drifted to the last time he'd seen his old friend. Jake had been a mess—out of shape, exhausted, constantly complaining about his health. Back then, David hadn't seen a way out for him. He had assumed Jake's struggles would swallow him whole.

But then... something had changed. The next time David saw him, Jake was almost unrecognizable—lean, confident, exuding a calm strength that hadn't been there before.

David had told himself it was just a phase. That Jake had probably jumped on some fitness craze that would fade like all the others. But Jake had kept going. Year after year. And David? He had let life happen to him.

His phone buzzed, jolting him back.

Jake: *"I was hoping you'd say that. Let's meet. Tomorrow. Noon. My place?"*

David's fingers hovered over the screen. Did he really want to do this? Seeing Jake again meant confronting everything he had been avoiding.

Another message came before he could overthink it.

Jake: *"No excuses, Carter. I've been where you are."*

David exhaled sharply. This wasn't the old Jake, the one who would've brushed things off with a joke or an easy out. No, this was a different man.

David: *"Alright. I'll be there."*

The next morning, David gripped the steering wheel tightly as he pulled into Jake's driveway. The house was different. The last time he had been here, the yard had been overgrown, the porch cluttered with forgotten projects. Now, everything was neat, the colors warm, the energy different.

The front door opened before he could knock.

Jake stood there, arms crossed, a knowing smile tugging at the corner of his mouth. He looked good—strong, relaxed, at peace in a way David didn't understand.

"Damn, Carter," Jake said, stepping forward. "Took you long enough."

David let out a dry chuckle. "Yeah, well... life happens."

Jake gave him a slow, assessing look—not judgmental, just observant. "Yeah. It does."

Inside, the air smelled fresh—lemons, maybe mint. It was subtle but invigorating. There was an energy in the space, something alive.

"You drink coffee?" Jake asked, already moving toward the kitchen.

David nodded. "Yeah, I—"

"Scratch that." Jake handed him a glass of water. "You drink this first."

David raised an eyebrow but took the glass. "What, you got rules now?"

Jake leaned against the counter, arms crossed. "Damn right. And rule number one—hydrate before anything else."

David smirked but took a sip. "So what is this? Some kind of health cult?"

Jake didn't laugh. Instead, he studied him for a beat before answering. "It's about taking control, Carter. Something I should've done years ago."

David's smirk faded. "You think I'm out of control?"

Jake didn't blink. "I think you've been surviving, not living."

The words landed harder than David expected. He set the glass down, rubbing the back of his neck. "Alright. So where do I start?"

Jake exhaled, his expression shifting into something more serious. "First, you figure out how you got here."

David frowned. "I know how. Stress, bad eating, no exercise..."

Jake shook his head. "That's just the surface. The real problem started before that."

David felt a chill creep down his spine. "Before?"

Jake nodded. "It's in your head, man. It's the way you've been thinking, the way you've been letting things slide. You don't just wake up one day and find yourself here. It happens slowly, and you let it happen."

David swallowed. He didn't like the way that sounded. "So what—you think this is all in my head?"

Jake tapped his temple. "Everything starts here. You can hit the gym, follow a meal plan, but if you don't fix this, none of it will stick."

David looked away, tension coiling in his chest. He had come for a pep talk, maybe some workout advice. Not... this.

Jake must have sensed his hesitation because his next words cut through the space between them.

"You want to fix this?" He took a step closer, his voice lower. "Then you need to ask yourself one thing."

David met his gaze, something uneasy twisting inside him. "What?"

Jake held his stare, the weight of the moment thick in the air.

"Are you willing to fight for your life?"

Silence stretched between them.

David's heart pounded.

He didn't have an answer.

Not yet.

Facing the Hard Truth

David stared at Jake, his stomach twisting into knots. *Are you willing to fight for your life?* The words echoed in his mind, louder than he wanted them to.

He had never thought of it that way. Sure, he had noticed the weight creeping on, the sluggishness, the aches that lingered longer than they used to. But fighting? That made it sound like he was in a battle.

Maybe he was.

He took a sip of the water Jake had given him, his throat dry. "I... I don't know."

Jake studied him for a moment, then nodded. "That's honest. And honesty is where it starts."

David exhaled, rubbing his hands over his face. "Man, I thought I was just here to get some workout tips, maybe a meal plan or something."

Jake smirked. "That's what most people think. They want a quick fix—some magic diet or workout plan that'll make everything better in a month. But you and I both know that's not how this works."

David sighed. "Yeah."

Jake walked over to a small cabinet and pulled out a journal, tossing it onto the kitchen counter in front of David.

"What's this?" David asked, eyeing the worn leather cover.

"My first journal from when I started my transformation," Jake said. "Open it."

David hesitated but flipped through the pages. The first few entries were scrawled in messy, frustrated handwriting.

Day 1: I feel like shit. My back hurts. My stomach is bigger than I thought. I don't even know where to start.

Day 2: Didn't want to work out today. I almost quit before I even started. But I went for a walk. Not much, but something.

David kept flipping, feeling an odd sense of connection with the words on the page.

Jake leaned against the counter. "See? It wasn't easy. I had to fight my way through every excuse, every doubt. I had to want it. And if you're not ready to want it, nothing I say or do will change that."

David closed the journal, his chest tight. He felt exposed, like Jake was holding a mirror up to his own struggles.

Jake crossed his arms. "So let's get real for a second. Why are you really here?"

David hesitated. "I told you. My doctor warned me—"

"No." Jake shook his head. "That's what pushed you here. But why are you here?"

David opened his mouth to argue but stopped. The truth sat heavy in his gut.

"I don't recognize myself anymore," he finally admitted. His voice was quiet, raw. "I wake up tired. My body aches in ways it never used to. I see Lisa looking at me with... concern. And I hate it."

Jake nodded slowly. "That's a start."

David clenched his jaw. "But I don't know if I have what it takes. What if it's too late?"

Jake's expression hardened. "That's bullshit."

David blinked. "Excuse me?"

"You heard me." Jake's voice was firm. "It's not too late. But if you keep telling yourself that, it will be. The only thing stopping you is your own damn mindset."

David's fingers curled into fists. A part of him wanted to argue, to push back, to tell Jake he didn't understand. But Jake did understand. He had been here before.

Silence stretched between them.

Jake finally spoke again, softer this time. "I'm not gonna sugarcoat this, Carter. It's going to suck. You're going to want to quit. Your body will fight you every step of the way at first. But I promise you, if you show up—every damn day—you'll see a difference."

David swallowed hard. "And if I fail?"

Jake's eyes locked onto his. "Then you get back up. And you keep fighting."

David exhaled sharply. His mind was spinning, but for the first time in a long time, he felt something stir inside him. A flicker of determination.

Jake smirked. "Now, finish your water. Your first test starts in five minutes."

David frowned. "Test?"

Jake's smirk widened. "Oh yeah. We're going for a run."

David's stomach dropped. "I haven't run in years."

Jake clapped him on the shoulder. "Good. Then this will be fun."

David groaned. What the hell did I just sign up for?

The First Step is the Hardest

David followed Jake outside, his heart pounding—not from exertion, but from dread. The morning air was crisp, a slight breeze cutting through the early sun. The neighborhood was quiet, except for the occasional chirp of birds or the distant hum of a lawnmower.

Jake stretched his arms over his head, looking perfectly at ease, while David stood stiff, trying to remember the last time he had done any kind of serious physical activity.

"Alright," Jake said, rolling his shoulders. "We're gonna start slow. Just a light jog."

David scoffed. "Jog? Man, I was expecting maybe some stretches or push-ups. I haven't run in years."

Jake grinned. "Exactly why we're starting with a run. No more talking. Let's go."

Before David could protest, Jake took off at a steady pace, glancing back over his shoulder. David hesitated, then reluctantly pushed himself forward, his legs feeling heavier than he remembered.

The first few strides weren't bad. His body recognized the motion, even if it had been years since he last ran. But by the time he reached the end of the block, his breathing was already labored.

Jake kept his pace steady. "Relax, Carter. Breathe in through your nose, out through your mouth."

David grunted in response, his chest tightening. His legs were already screaming at him. His stomach felt like a lead weight.

They turned the corner, and suddenly, the road stretched longer than David wanted to admit. He slowed down instinctively, hands on his hips, gasping.

Jake jogged back to him. "No stopping. Keep moving."

David shot him a glare. "Easy for you to say."

Jake chuckled. "You're not gonna die, man. You just need to push past that voice in your head telling you to quit."

David wiped the sweat from his brow. He hadn't even run for five minutes, and he already felt like collapsing.

Jake clapped him on the shoulder. "Look, you're out here. That's step one. Most guys in your position would still be sitting on the couch, convincing themselves they'll start 'tomorrow.'"

David let out a dry laugh. "Yeah, well, tomorrow sounds a lot better than right now."

Jake smirked. "Too bad. We're here now."

David groaned, forcing himself to start moving again. His muscles protested, but he kept going. Step by step.

A few houses down, a woman in her 60s power-walked past them, nodding with a friendly smile. "Morning, boys."

David barely managed a nod back. Jake, of course, responded with a full grin. "Morning, Linda."

As she passed, Jake chuckled. "See? Linda's out here getting it done. No excuses."

David muttered under his breath. "Linda probably didn't eat a double cheeseburger last night."

Jake grinned. "Probably not. But hey, that's why we're doing this."

David wanted to quit. Every part of him was screaming to stop. But something about Jake's relentless attitude kept him moving.

They turned another corner, and David's feet felt like cinder blocks.

Jake glanced at him. "Almost there. Just one more block."

David huffed. "You keep saying that."

Jake smirked. "You're catching on."

With a determined grunt, David forced himself forward, step by step, breath by breath. His lungs burned, his legs ached, but he wasn't stopping.

Finally, Jake slowed to a walk, and David followed, nearly collapsing on the sidewalk. He bent over, hands on his knees, gasping for air.

Jake gave him a nod. "Not bad for your first day."

David glared up at him. "I feel like I'm gonna puke."

Jake chuckled. "That's how you know you did it right."

David groaned, shaking his head. But somewhere deep inside, buried under the exhaustion, he felt something else.

A flicker of pride.

He had survived.

Maybe—just maybe—he could do this.

But then Jake said something that made his stomach drop all over again.

"Alright, Carter. Now let's talk about your diet."

David groaned. "Oh, come on, man. Let me have this moment."

Jake laughed. "No time to celebrate. This is just the beginning."

David shook his head, exhaling. He had a feeling this was going to be harder than he thought.

HEALING ME NOW

The Truth About Food

David sat at Jake's kitchen counter, still catching his breath from the run. His shirt clung to his sweaty back, and his legs felt like they'd been replaced with bricks. He wanted to collapse onto the couch and never move again, but he had a feeling Jake wouldn't let him.

Jake placed a plate in front of him—grilled chicken, avocado slices, and steamed broccoli.

David frowned. "Where's the bread? The potatoes? The sauce?"

Jake smirked. "Gone. Welcome to your new diet."

David groaned. "Man, you're really not going easy on me, huh?"

Jake sat across from him, a glass of water in hand. "Nope. Because your biggest enemy isn't just inactivity. It's what you put in your body."

David picked up a fork and stabbed a piece of chicken. "I thought running was bad. But taking away my burgers? My fries? That's just cruel."

Jake chuckled. "Look, I'm not saying you can never eat that stuff again. But right now? Your body is inflamed, your metabolism is sluggish, and your energy levels are crashing because of what you're fueling yourself with."

David sighed. "Alright, professor. Break it down for me."

Jake leaned back. "Simple. Food is fuel. You wouldn't put cheap, low-grade gas in a high-performance car and expect it to run smoothly, right?"

David raised an eyebrow. "Hate to break it to you, but I'm not exactly a high-performance anything right now."

Jake smirked. "Yet. But we're changing that."

David took a bite of the chicken. It was surprisingly good. Simple, but good. He chewed thoughtfully. "So what's the game plan?"

Jake nodded. "For now, you're going to stick to whole, unprocessed foods. Lean proteins, healthy fats, and complex carbs in moderation. No added sugars, no junk, no alcohol."

David nearly choked. "Wait—no *beer*?"

Jake shook his head. "Not if you're serious about this."

David groaned. "Damn. You really are trying to kill me."

Jake laughed. "No, I'm trying to keep you alive."

David sighed, poking at the avocado on his plate. "So, what happens if I mess up?"

Jake shrugged. "You will. Everyone does. It's not about being perfect. It's about consistency."

David thought about that as he took another bite. He'd spent years in a cycle of bad habits. If he wanted to break them, he'd have to push past the discomfort, the cravings, the old mindset that told him he was too far gone.

Jake stood up, stretching. "Alright, Carter. You survived your first run, you're eating your first clean meal. Now comes the real test."

David frowned. "What's that?"

Jake grinned. "Sticking to it."

David exhaled. He had a long road ahead. But for the first time in years, he felt something stir inside him.

Hope. And maybe, just maybe... a little bit of determination.

CHAPTER 2

THE RESISTANCE BEGINS

The First Temptation

David woke up the next morning feeling like he had been hit by a truck. Every muscle in his body ached, from his calves to his shoulders. Even shifting in bed sent a dull pain radiating through his legs.

"What the hell did I sign up for?" he thought, wincing as he swung his feet onto the floor.

His phone buzzed.

Jake: *"Morning, Carter. Hydrate. Then stretch. Then eat. No skipping steps."*

David rolled his eyes but reached for the glass of water on his nightstand. He had to admit, yesterday had been eye-opening. It wasn't just the run—it was the realization that he had been lying to himself for years.

But knowing he needed to change and actually doing it? Those were two different things.

Downstairs, Lisa was already in the kitchen. The smell of coffee and toast filled the air, and David's stomach rumbled.

"Hey," she said, glancing at him over her mug. "How was your run?"

David groaned, stretching his back. "Brutal. I think I left part of my soul on the sidewalk."

Lisa chuckled. "Good. Maybe you'll find it again tomorrow."

He smirked. "Very funny."

She placed a plate on the table—scrambled eggs, toast, and butter. His usual breakfast. The smell was *incredible*.

But he hesitated. Jake's words from yesterday echoed in his mind. *No added sugars. No junk.* He had eaten clean for one meal, but now, staring at the buttered toast, his cravings kicked in full force.

Lisa noticed his hesitation. "What's wrong?"

David sighed. "Jake's got me on some kind of clean-eating thing. No processed food. No bread."

Lisa arched an eyebrow. "You love bread."

"I *know*," David muttered, rubbing his face.

She slid the plate closer. "It's just toast, Dave."

It *was* just toast. And yet, it wasn't. He had always found excuses to bend the rules, to cheat "just a little." A skipped workout here, an unhealthy meal there. It had all added up.

He looked at Lisa, then at the toast.

Then, with a deep breath, he pushed the plate back.

"I think I'll make some eggs and avocado instead."

Lisa's eyes widened. "Seriously?"

David stood up, heading to the fridge. "Yeah. Seriously."

As he cracked eggs into the pan, something strange happened. He felt... proud.

It was just a small decision. But maybe small decisions were where the real battles were won.

Jake had been right. The real challenge wasn't the run. It was *this*.

Resisting the old habits. Choosing better.

One meal at a time.

Old Habits Die Hard

David sat at the kitchen table, eating his eggs and avocado, still feeling the ghost of temptation whispering in his ear. The toast had smelled so good. He knew it wouldn't have killed him to eat it. One slice, no big deal, right?

But that was the trap. The same one he had fallen into a thousand times before. Just this once turned into just one more—and before he knew it, he was back in the same cycle.

Lisa sipped her coffee, watching him with amusement. "I'm impressed."

David smirked. "Yeah, yeah. I know. No toast today. Let's see if I survive."

Lisa laughed. "I wasn't talking about the toast. I mean the fact that you're actually committing to this. It's been a long time since I've seen you this serious about something."

David shrugged. "It's only been a day."

"But you want it," Lisa said, leaning forward. "And that's different."

David nodded slowly, letting the words settle. She was right. He did want it. But wanting wasn't enough—he had learned that the hard way.

The real test came when life threw obstacles in the way.

And, as if the universe was listening, his phone buzzed.

Work Group Chat:
◈ Friday Happy Hour at Miller's! Beers & Burgers on the boss! ◈

David groaned. Just great. The guys at work loved their Friday outings—cheap beer, greasy food, and hours of complaining about the job.

Lisa saw the look on his face. "What is it?"

He turned the phone toward her.

She winced. "Oof. That's rough timing."

David sighed. "Tell me about it."

A week ago, he wouldn't have thought twice about it. But now? He was barely twenty-four hours into this change. Could he really sit there, surrounded by burgers, fries, and cold beer, and not cave?

Lisa set her mug down. "You know, you don't have to go."

David ran a hand through his hair. "Yeah, but if I skip, I'm gonna hear about it all week. 'Carter's too good for burgers now.'"

Lisa tilted her head. "Or... you could go and prove to yourself that you can stick with this, even when it's hard."

David sighed, rubbing his temples. "I don't know, Lisa. It's just—"

His phone buzzed again.

Jake: "Remember what I said: The fight isn't in the gym. It's in the choices you make every day."

David stared at the message. He exhaled sharply.

Lisa smirked. "Let me guess. Jake?"

David nodded. "Yeah. The guy's like a damn mind reader."

She chuckled. "So? What's the plan?"

David thought about it. He could make excuses, skip the happy hour, and avoid temptation altogether. But that wouldn't help in the long run.

If he was going to really change, he had to be able to live his life without falling into old habits.

He took a deep breath and texted back in the group chat.

David: "I'll be there. But no beer for me."

A flood of laughing emojis popped up immediately.

Mike: "Who are you and what have you done with Carter??"

Tom: "Carter's on a diet!! ◇"

Boss: "More beer for the rest of us, then. See you there."

David locked his phone and slid it onto the table.

Lisa raised an eyebrow. "Brave move."

David smirked, standing up. "We'll see how brave I feel when I'm sitting in front of a plate of wings."

She grinned. "Good luck."

David exhaled and stretched his sore legs.

One meal down.

One temptation avoided. Now, onto the next battle.

MARK FLORY

The Happy Hour Test

The sun was beginning to set as David pulled into the parking lot of Miller's, the familiar neon sign flickering above the entrance. Friday happy hour was already in full swing, the muffled roar of laughter and conversation spilling out into the evening air.

He gripped the steering wheel, inhaling deeply. *You got this. Just don't cave.*

With a final exhale, he stepped out of the car and headed inside.

The smell of sizzling burgers and fried appetizers hit him immediately. His stomach clenched. *Damn it, that smells good.* He shook it off and walked toward the usual table in the back.

"Look who actually showed up!" Mike, one of his coworkers, grinned as David approached. "We thought you turned into a health nut overnight and forgot about us."

David smirked. "Not quite."

Tom, another coworker, lifted his beer. "Well, we'll see how long that lasts."

David slid into a seat and grabbed a menu. He wasn't about to order a salad and let them tear him apart for it, but he also wasn't going to go back on his commitment.

A waitress walked up, pen poised. "What can I get you, Dave?"

He glanced at the menu. The cheeseburger stared back at him like an old friend. *Just one bite*, a voice in his head whispered.

He cleared his throat. "Grilled chicken, no bun. Side of veggies instead of fries."

The table went silent for half a second before Mike snorted. "What the hell did Jake do to you?"

David chuckled. "Just making better choices, that's all."

Tom shook his head. "Better choices? Bro, we come here to forget about choices."

The waitress smiled, jotting down the order. "I think it's great. Anything to drink?"

David hesitated, then made the call. "Just water."

Mike groaned dramatically. "Carter, you are ruining the tradition."

David smirked. "Relax, Mike. I'm still here, aren't I?"

Tom leaned back. "Alright, serious question. What's the end goal here? You trying to get ripped? Run a marathon?"

David exhaled, running a hand through his hair. "I just... I don't like where I'm at. I feel slow, and tired all the time. My doctor gave me a wake-up call, and honestly? I don't want to wait until it's too late."

A brief silence followed.

Then Mike raised his beer. "Alright, then. To Carter, for at least trying to outlive the rest of us."

The table laughed, and David clinked his water glass against their drinks.

For the first time in a long time, he felt in control.

But just as he started to relax, Tom grinned and waved the waitress back over.

"Alright, fine, Carter. No beer. No fries. But let's see how strong your willpower really is."

David frowned. "What are you talking about?"

Tom's grin widened. "One order of wings. Extra spicy."

David's stomach dropped.
Oh, hell.

The Wings Showdown

David stared at Tom, then at the waitress, who was already jotting down the order with a smirk.

"Coming right up," she said, before disappearing toward the kitchen.

David exhaled slowly. Alright, stay calm. It's just wings.

Tom leaned forward, grinning. "So, what's the move, Carter? You gonna resist the greatest temptation known to man?"

Mike laughed. "Oh man, I love this. Carter's first real test."

David smirked, shaking his head. "You guys are acting like I just joined a monastery."

"Close enough," Mike said, sipping his beer. "No booze, no fries, no bread... Now, no wings?"

David leaned back in his chair, considering his options. He wasn't against eating wings. Hell, they were technically protein. But he knew these weren't just wings—they were deep-fried, doused in sauce, and loaded with who knew how much sugar and sodium.

This wasn't about one meal. It was about proving to himself that he could make the right choice, even when it sucked.

The waitress returned, setting a massive basket of steaming, bright red buffalo wings in the middle of the table. The scent hit David like a punch to the gut.

Mike grabbed one immediately, took a bite, and groaned in pleasure. "Damn, these hit different today."

Tom picked one up, waving it in David's face. "Come on, man. Just one. No one's gonna judge you."

David stared at it. His body wanted it. His taste buds were practically begging.

Then he heard Jake's voice in his head. The fight isn't in the gym. It's in the choices you make every day.

With a slow exhale, David shook his head. "Nah. I'm good."

Tom's jaw dropped. "Seriously?"

David nodded, picking up his fork and digging into his grilled chicken. "Yeah. I told myself I was going to stick to this. That's what I'm doing."

Mike whistled. "Damn. Never thought I'd see the day."

Tom shook his head but laughed. "Alright, fine. But just so you know, you missed out on heaven."

David smirked, taking another bite of his meal.

It wasn't heaven.

But it was control.

And right now? That tasted even better.

Breaking the Cycle

As the night went on, David realized something surprising—he was actually *having fun*.

At first, he had braced himself for the usual peer pressure, expecting Mike and Tom to ride him the whole time. But after the initial shock of his food choices wore off, the conversation drifted back to normal.

They joked about work, argued about football, and swapped ridiculous stories about their younger days.

And for the first time in a long time, David wasn't just *there*. He was *present*.

No brain fog. No sluggishness from a heavy meal. No guilt weighing him down.

So this is what it feels like to actually take care of myself.

He almost laughed at the thought.

When was the last time he had left happy hour *not* feeling bloated, tired, or guilty about what he'd eaten?

Maybe this whole "self-discipline" thing wasn't so bad after all.

As the group started to wrap up, Tom leaned back in his chair, rubbing his stomach. "Alright, I'll admit it. I feel like *garbage* right now."

Mike groaned. "Same. Why do we do this every week?"

David smirked. "Because it's tradition?"

Tom sighed. "Yeah, well, maybe I need a *new* tradition."

David raised an eyebrow. "You saying you want to get on the Carter health plan?"

Tom scoffed. "Let's not get ahead of ourselves. But I *am* saying... maybe you're onto something."

David was about to respond when his phone buzzed.

Jake: *"How'd it go?"*

David smirked and typed back: **"Survived. No beer, no fries, no wings."**

Jake's reply came almost instantly.

Jake: *"Damn. Who are you and what have you done with the real Carter?"*

David chuckled, shaking his head.

He wasn't sure who he was turning into yet.

But for the first time in a long time, he was excited to find out.

CHAPTER 3

PUSHING THE LIMIT

The Wake-Up Call—Round Two

David groaned as his alarm blared at 5:30 AM. His body screamed in protest, sore in places he hadn't even known could be sore. Every muscle ached from the previous day's run, and his stomach grumbled, reminding him that he'd skipped the usual late-night snack.

Is this what progress feels like?

He shut off the alarm, rolled onto his back, and stared at the ceiling.

His old self would have hit snooze—maybe even skipped the whole workout. But something was different this time.

The commitment he had made at happy hour still lingered in his mind. He had passed the first real test of temptation. Now, he had to prove to himself that it wasn't a fluke.

His phone buzzed.

Jake: *"Rise and shine, Carter. We're running at six."*

David exhaled sharply. *Of course we are.*

Dragging himself out of bed, he pulled on his sneakers and trudged to the bathroom. His reflection caught his eye. He looked tired, sure—but there was something else.

Something he hadn't seen in a long time.

Determination.

The morning air was crisp as David pulled up to the park where Jake was waiting. His friend looked like he had been up for hours, stretching and jogging in place.

David groaned. "How do you have this much energy already?"

Jake grinned. "It's called discipline, Carter. You'll get there."

David rolled his eyes. "Yeah, yeah. Let's just get this over with."

Jake laughed. "Oh, no, my friend. Today's not about 'getting it over with.'"

David frowned. "What do you mean?"

Jake clapped him on the back. "Today, we push limits."

David's stomach dropped. "That... doesn't sound good."

Jake smirked. "Depends on your definition of 'good.'"

David groaned, already regretting waking up.

This was going to hurt.

The Test of Endurance

David stretched his legs, already regretting his life choices. The park was quiet except for the occasional jogger and the distant sound of birds waking up. The air was crisp, the kind that normally made him want to wrap himself in a blanket and go back to sleep.

Jake, on the other hand, looked far too excited for this early in the morning.

"Alright, Carter," Jake said, cracking his knuckles. "Yesterday was just a warm-up. Today, we're stepping it up."

David groaned. "Jake, I barely survived yesterday. What do you mean *stepping it up*?"

Jake smirked. "We're adding intervals. Short bursts of speed between steady jogging. It'll improve endurance, burn fat, and wake your body up faster."

David sighed. "Can't I just do another slow jog? I *like* slow jogs."

Jake shook his head. "Nope. Growth happens when you push past comfort. You're too comfortable, Carter. That's how you ended up here."

David rubbed his face. He hated that Jake was right.

"Fine," he grumbled. "What's the plan?"

Jake clapped his hands. "We jog at a steady pace for two minutes, then sprint for thirty seconds. Repeat that for twenty minutes."

David blinked. "Sprint? For thirty whole seconds?"

Jake chuckled. "It's not that bad. Just try to keep up."

David exhaled. "Let's get this over with."

They started at an easy pace, David's legs still stiff from the last run. But after a few minutes, he found a rhythm. The soreness dulled, and the steady movement became… tolerable.

Then Jake picked up the pace.

"Alright, Carter—sprint!"

David gritted his teeth and pushed forward, his feet pounding the pavement. His lungs burned, his muscles protested, and after what felt like an eternity, Jake finally called, "Back to jogging!"

David nearly collapsed.

"That—" he gasped, "—was awful."

Jake laughed. "That was *one* round. We've got nine more."

David groaned, wiping sweat from his forehead.

What the hell did I sign up for?

Fighting Through the Pain

David's lungs felt like they were on fire. His legs burned, his arms were heavy, and sweat dripped down his forehead like he'd just walked through a rainstorm.

And they were only halfway through.

"Come on, Carter!" Jake called out, barely winded. "Two more minutes of steady jog, then we sprint again!"

David groaned, dragging his feet forward. His body screamed at him to stop, to collapse on the grass and never move again. But a small, stubborn part of him refused to quit.

He wasn't going back to the old version of himself.

"Alright!" Jake shouted. "Sprint—now!"

David clenched his fists and pushed forward. His legs wobbled, his breath came in short, ragged gasps, but he kept going.

Fifteen seconds.

Twenty seconds.

His vision blurred slightly, and his chest tightened.

Then—finally—Jake's voice cut through the pounding in his ears.

"Jog!"

David slowed down, barely holding himself together. His feet felt like bricks.

Jake clapped him on the back. "Good. That was better."

David shot him a look. "Better? I think I'm dying."

Jake laughed. "Nah. That's just your body waking up."

David wiped the sweat from his face, shaking his head. "If this is what waking up feels like, I might prefer staying asleep."

Jake smirked. "Yeah, but asleep is how you got here."

David swallowed hard. He *hated* how right Jake was.

Another minute passed, and Jake called out, "Last sprint. Dig deep, Carter. Let's go!"

David wanted to argue. His legs were barely functioning. His whole body screamed *no more.*

But something in him snapped.

With a growl, he pushed forward, running faster than before. His arms pumped, his legs churned, and for a brief moment—despite the pain—he felt *alive.*

Thirty seconds later, he slowed, gasping, his hands on his knees. His heart pounded, but a small smile crept onto his face.

Jake nodded. "That's what I'm talking about."

David shook his head. "That... was hell."

Jake chuckled. "Yeah. But you survived."

David exhaled, straightening up. He had survived. And tomorrow, he'd do it again.

Because for the first time in a long time, he wasn't running from something.

He was running *toward* something.

The Aftermath

David collapsed onto a park bench, his legs trembling, his lungs still working overtime. His shirt clung to his back, drenched in sweat, and his heart hammered in his chest like it was trying to break free.

Jake, of course, barely looked tired. He was breathing hard, sure, but he wasn't hunched over like a man who had just run for his life.

David wiped his face with his sleeve. "You know... there's a fine line between pushing limits and attempted murder."

Jake grinned. "You didn't die, did you?"

David glared at him. "Debatable."

Jake chuckled and tossed him a bottle of water. "Drink. Hydration is key."

David twisted off the cap and took a long gulp, letting the cool liquid soothe his throat. His muscles still felt like jelly, but somewhere deep inside, there was a flicker of something else.

Pride.

He had done it.

Not perfectly. Not easily. But he had pushed through when everything in him screamed to stop.

And that meant something.

Jake sat down next to him, stretching out his legs. "You know, most guys in your position wouldn't have finished that."

David snorted. "Gee, thanks for the vote of confidence."

Jake shook his head. "I'm serious. I've trained guys who gave up halfway through their first workout. Said it was 'too much' or that they 'weren't built for it.' But you kept going."

David exhaled, rolling his shoulders. "Yeah. Because I don't want to be that guy anymore."

Jake nodded. "Good. Because this? This is just the beginning."

David sighed. "Yeah, yeah. I figured."

A comfortable silence settled between them as they watched the early morning runners pass by.

Then Jake stood up, clapping his hands together. "Alright. Go home, eat something with protein, and rest. Tomorrow, we hit the gym."

David groaned. "I hate you."

Jake laughed. "Nah, you don't. You just hate the work."

David smirked. "Fine. I *strongly dislike* you."

Jake grinned. "I'll take it."

David stood up, his legs still shaky, but his mind clearer than it had been in years.

Tomorrow, the gym.

And for the first time, he wasn't dreading it.

He was ready.

MARK FLORY

Welcome to the Gym

David pulled into the gym parking lot the next morning, gripping the steering wheel tighter than necessary. His body was *still* sore from the run, but it wasn't just the physical pain making him hesitate.

It was *this place*.

The gym.

Once upon a time, he had practically *lived* in places like this. Back when he was younger, stronger, and when working out was second nature. But that was years ago.

Now?

Now he was the out-of-shape guy walking into a place full of fit people who never let themselves slide.

His phone buzzed.

Jake: *"Don't sit in your car overthinking it. I see you."*

David snapped his head up. Sure enough, Jake was leaning against the entrance, smirking at him through the glass doors.

David groaned. "Of course he saw me."

With a sigh, he grabbed his water bottle, climbed out of the car, and trudged toward the entrance.

Jake clapped him on the shoulder as he walked in. "You look thrilled to be here."

David rolled his eyes. "Oh yeah, this is my *dream* morning."

Jake laughed, leading him inside. "Relax. No one's judging you. Everyone here started somewhere."

David glanced around. The gym was alive with movement—weights clanking, treadmills humming, people grunting through reps. It was overwhelming.

Jake seemed to read his mind. "You're not here to impress anyone, Carter. You're here to get better."

David exhaled. "Alright. What's the plan?"

Jake grinned. "Leg day."

David froze. "Wait, *what*?"

Jake patted him on the back. "Oh yeah. We're starting strong."

David groaned. "I take back everything. I *definitely* hate you."

Jake laughed, already leading him toward the squat racks.

This was going to hurt.

THE PAIN OF PROGRESS

Leg Day Hell

David stood in front of the squat rack, staring at the bar like it was his mortal enemy.

Leg day.

Of *course* Jake started him with leg day.

Jake stood beside him, arms crossed, looking far too smug. "Alright, Carter. Time to see what those legs can do."

David exhaled sharply. "What if I told you my legs are *still* recovering from that run?"

Jake smirked. "Then I'd tell you this is exactly why we're doing this."

David groaned but stepped forward. The last time he had done squats, he had been in his prime—strong, confident, a regular at the gym. Now? He felt like a stranger in his own body.

Jake adjusted the weight. "We'll start light. Focus on form. Feet shoulder-width apart, core tight, drop low, and drive up."

David nodded, took his position, and gripped the bar. As he lowered himself into the first squat, his legs immediately screamed in protest.

Jake chuckled. "Feel that?"

David gritted his teeth as he pushed back up. "Oh yeah. I feel *everything*."

"Good. That's your muscles waking up."

David rolled his eyes. "Pretty sure they're *dying*, not waking up."

Jake laughed. "Nah, they're just pissed at you. Keep going."

Rep after rep, the burn intensified. By the time he hit his tenth squat, sweat was dripping down his face, and his legs were trembling.

He racked the bar and exhaled sharply, hands on his knees. "Holy *hell*."

Jake grinned. "Welcome back to the gym."

David shook his head. "I hate this."

Jake clapped him on the back. "No, you hate how weak you feel. But that's temporary."

David groaned as he stood up straight. "Temporary, huh? So when does it stop hurting?"

Jake smirked. "Give it a few weeks."

David blinked. "*Weeks*?"

Jake chuckled. "Hey, you signed up for this."

David exhaled and shook out his legs.

Leg day was hell.

But deep down, buried under the soreness, was something else.

Satisfaction.

Because he had shown up.

And that? That was a win.

When Every Step Hurts

David hobbled toward the gym exit, every step feeling like a punishment. His legs were officially useless. If he had to run for his life right now, he'd just accept his fate.

Jake walked beside him, looking far too *not* in pain. "How're we feeling?"

David shot him a look. "Like I got hit by a truck. And then the truck backed up and ran me over again for fun."

Jake laughed. "Yeah, that sounds about right."

David gripped the doorframe as they stepped outside. "How do people *like* this?"

Jake smirked. "They don't like the pain. They like what comes *after*."

David sighed, stretching his leg, immediately regretting it. "What comes after?"

Jake tossed him a protein shake. "Strength. Endurance. Confidence. You'll see."

David cracked open the bottle and took a long sip. His body needed it, but his mind was still fighting him.

He had shown up. He had done the work. But the soreness? It was already settling in, and he knew tomorrow would be even worse.

Jake clapped him on the shoulder. "The real test is tomorrow."

David frowned. "What do you mean?"

Jake grinned. "Showing up when you're sore."

David groaned. "Are you kidding? I'm gonna need a wheelchair."

Jake chuckled. "Nope. You're gonna stretch, hydrate, and come back for more."

David exhaled. He knew Jake was right. If he quit now, it'd be just like all the other times.

But he was done quitting.

Even if it meant limping his way forward.

The Morning After

David knew it was going to be bad.

But he hadn't expected *this*.

The second he tried to move, a sharp pain shot through his legs, locking him in place. He groaned, flopping back onto the bed, staring at the ceiling.

I am never getting up again.

Lisa's laughter drifted in from the doorway. "I take it leg day went well?"

David turned his head slowly, shooting her a glare. "Define 'well.'"

She smirked, crossing her arms. "You look like you got into a fight with a staircase and lost."

David sighed. "It *feels* like I lost."

Lisa walked over, sitting on the edge of the bed. "So... are you going back today?"

David groaned. "Jake expects me to. But I can barely move. How does he think I'm gonna work out when I can't even stand?"

Lisa smiled. "I think that's the point."

David frowned. "What do you mean?"

She nudged him gently. "He's testing you. Seeing if you'll push through or fall back into old habits."

David exhaled. He hated how right she was.

Lisa stood up, stretching. "Besides, I read somewhere that moving *helps* sore muscles."

David scoffed. "Moving is what *got* me into this mess."

Lisa grinned. "And moving is what'll get you out of it."

David let out a long breath. His body wanted to stay in bed forever.

But his mind?

His mind was telling him to get up.

Slowly, painfully, he rolled onto his side and swung his legs over the bed. His muscles screamed in protest, but he clenched his jaw and pushed through.

Lisa raised an eyebrow. "So, you're going?"

David stood up—wobbling like a newborn deer—and nodded. "Yeah."

Lisa smiled. "Proud of you."

David grabbed his phone, texting Jake.

David: *"You win. I'm coming."*

Jake's reply was instant.

Jake: *"Damn right you are. See you in 30."*

David sighed, already regretting everything.

But deep down, he knew—this was the moment that mattered.

Not the easy days.

Not the first workout.

The choice to keep going, even when it sucked.

And that? That's what was going to change him.

Pushing Through the Soreness

David gritted his teeth as he stepped into the gym, every muscle in his legs screaming in protest. Walking from the parking lot had been an ordeal. Climbing the single step at the entrance? Damn near impossible.

Jake was already inside, waiting near the free weights with that smug *I-told-you-this-would-hurt* look on his face.

"You actually showed up," Jake said, crossing his arms. "Didn't think you had it in you."

David exhaled sharply. "Trust me, neither did I."

Jake smirked. "How bad?"

David groaned, stretching his legs slightly. "Let's just say if someone pushed me over right now, I wouldn't get back up."

Jake laughed. "Good. That means you actually did the work yesterday."

David rolled his eyes. "Yeah, yeah. What's the plan today? Upper body? Please tell me it's upper body."

Jake nodded. "It is. But first..."

David's stomach dropped. "First *what?*"

Jake pointed toward the treadmill. "Ten minutes. Light jog."

David nearly cursed out loud. "Are you *serious*? My legs are barely functional!"

Jake grinned. "Exactly why you need to move them. Blood flow helps soreness. Trust me, you'll feel better after."

David let out a long, pained sigh. "You and I have *very* different definitions of 'better.'"

Jake chuckled. "Quit stalling, Carter. Let's go."

Muttering under his breath, David trudged toward the treadmill and climbed on. His legs resisted every movement, but he pressed start and forced himself into a slow, pathetic jog.

It sucked.

The first thirty seconds were brutal. Every step sent a dull ache through his thighs and calves. He clenched his jaw, trying not to limp, but the soreness was relentless.

But then... something strange happened.

After a couple of minutes, the stiffness started to fade. The tightness in his muscles loosened, and his legs—while still sore—became more *functional*.

Jake gave him a thumbs-up from across the gym. "Told you!"

David shook his head. "Still hate you!"

Jake grinned. "Good! That means I'm doing my job."

By the time the ten minutes were up, David was sweating but moving far better than before.

He slowed the treadmill to a walk, taking a deep breath.

Maybe Jake was right.

Maybe pushing through *was* the key.

Jake clapped him on the shoulder as he walked by. "Alright, now that your legs aren't made of cement, let's build some muscle."

David smirked, stepping off the treadmill.

"Finally. Something I *might* actually enjoy."

Jake chuckled. "We'll see about that."

David exhaled, rolling his shoulders.

Day two.

He was still in the fight.

And for the first time in a long time, he *wanted* to keep going.

Strength Over Struggle

David stood in front of the dumbbells, rolling his shoulders. His legs were still sore, but after the treadmill warm-up, they were at least semi-functional.

Jake grabbed a pair of dumbbells and nodded toward the bench. "Alright, Carter. Today, we hit the upper body. We're starting with bench press."

David smirked. "Finally, something that doesn't involve running."

Jake chuckled. "Don't get too excited. We're still working."

David settled onto the bench as Jake loaded up the bar. He gripped the steel, feeling its cold weight in his hands. It had been years since he'd done a proper bench press, but muscle memory was a funny thing.

"Alright," Jake said. "Controlled reps. No bouncing. No ego lifting. We're building strength, not showing off."

David exhaled and unracked the bar. As he lowered it, his arms trembled slightly—not from the weight, but from disuse. He pushed up, gritting his teeth.

It wasn't *easy*, but it wasn't impossible either.

Jake nodded in approval. "Good. Steady. Don't rush it."

Rep after rep, David felt his muscles waking up. His arms burned, his chest tightened, but he kept going.

By the time he racked the bar, his arms were shaking.

Jake grinned. "Welcome back to lifting."

David wiped the sweat from his forehead. "Forgot how much I missed this."

Jake smirked. "That's what they all say—until tomorrow when your arms don't work."

David groaned. "Great. Something to look forward to."

Jake tossed him a towel. "Progress hurts. But pain is temporary. Strength is permanent."

David let those words sink in.

He was tired. Sore. Struggling.

But for the first time in years, he was *getting stronger*.

And that? That was worth every drop of sweat.

CHAPTER 5

THE BREAKING POINT

When Doubt Creeps In

David collapsed onto his couch, arms limp at his sides, his entire body screaming in protest. The soreness wasn't just in his legs anymore—his chest, shoulders, and arms felt like they'd been through a war.

Lisa walked in from the kitchen, holding a mug of tea. She raised an eyebrow. "So, I take it the gym was a success?"

David groaned. "Define 'success.' If it means barely being able to lift my arms, then yeah. Huge success."

Lisa smirked. "Jake's really putting you through it, huh?"

David exhaled. "Oh, he's *loving* it."

She sat down beside him, setting her mug on the table. "You gonna keep going?"

David hesitated.

Was he?

He *wanted* to.

But his body was rebelling. The idea of waking up and doing it all again tomorrow felt overwhelming.

Lisa studied him for a moment. "You're thinking about quitting."

David frowned. "I didn't say that."

"You didn't have to." She nudged him. "It's written all over your face."

He sighed, staring at the ceiling. "It's just... I don't know if I can keep this up. Every workout feels like a fight. What if I just don't have it in me anymore?"

Lisa was quiet for a moment. Then she leaned forward. "You remember when you taught our nephew how to ride a bike?"

David frowned. "Yeah... what about it?"

"He fell about a dozen times. Skinned his knee twice. At one point, he sat on the curb and cried because he was *convinced* he'd never get it." She smiled. "But you told him the only way he'd fail is if he gave up."

David swallowed hard.

Lisa squeezed his arm. "You're that kid right now, David. And you have two choices—sit on the curb, or get back on the bike."

David exhaled slowly.

He knew she was right.

But that didn't make it any easier.

A Crossroads

David sat in silence, Lisa's words settling over him like a heavy weight.

Sit on the curb, or get back on the bike.

It sounded so simple.

But the exhaustion in his bones told a different story.

Lisa stood up, stretching. "You don't have to decide tonight. But I think you already know what you need to do."

David sighed as she walked back to the kitchen. Did he know?

His phone buzzed on the coffee table.

Jake: *"Feeling sore yet?"*

David smirked despite himself. *The man never stops.*

David: *"Sore isn't the word. More like completely wrecked."*

Jake: *"Good. That means it's working."*

David shook his head. The guy had a way of making misery sound like an achievement.

His phone buzzed again.

Jake: *"Listen, man. This is where most people quit. They feel the pain, they doubt themselves, and they slide back into old habits. But that's not you. Not this time."*

David swallowed hard.

Jake was right.

Lisa was right.

But *knowing* wasn't the same as *doing*.

His eyes drifted toward the hallway, where the bed was calling to him. Sleep sounded like the best plan right now. Maybe tomorrow, things would be clearer.

He was about to set his phone down when one last message came through.

Jake: *"We're hitting the gym at 6 AM. You in?"*

David stared at the screen.

This was it.

The moment that would decide everything.

He could ignore the message, sleep in, and let this whole thing slip away.

Or—

He could show up.

His fingers hovered over the keyboard for a long moment.

Then, slowly, he typed.

David: *"See you at 6."*

He let out a long breath.

There.

Decision made.

No turning back.

The Hardest Morning Yet

The blaring alarm at 5:30 AM felt like a personal attack.

David groaned, rolling onto his side, every muscle in his body protesting. His arms ached from yesterday's workout, his legs still burned from the first run, and his body screamed at him to stay in bed.

Maybe I should skip just this one time.

The thought crept in, tempting, logical. It was just one day. He could start again tomorrow, right?

Then he remembered his own words to Jake. *See you at 6.*

David exhaled, forcing himself to sit up.

No turning back.

His body was sluggish as he got dressed, his limbs heavy, his mind still foggy from sleep.

Lisa stirred beside him, blinking groggily. "You're actually going?"

David smirked, rubbing his sore shoulder. "Apparently."

She smiled. "Proud of you."

That alone was enough to push him forward.

The gym parking lot was nearly empty when he pulled in. The sky was still dark, the air crisp. For a brief moment, he sat in the driver's seat, gripping the wheel.

Then Jake appeared, knocking on the window.

David sighed and rolled it down. "You always do this?"

Jake grinned. "Do what?"

"Stand outside like some kind of motivational gym gremlin?"

Jake laughed. "Only for the ones who need it most."

David shook his head, climbing out of the car. His muscles groaned in protest, but he ignored them.

Jake clapped him on the back. "You showed up. That's half the battle."

David stretched his arms, wincing. "And the other half?"

Jake smirked. "The part where we make you regret showing up."

David groaned. "Why do I feel like I walked into a trap?"

Jake led the way inside. "Because you did."

David exhaled.

This was going to suck.

But he was here.

And that meant he was still in the fight.

Pushing Past the Wall

The gym smelled like rubber mats, sweat, and metal. The early morning crowd was sparse—just a few dedicated lifters and the occasional runner on a treadmill.

Jake led David toward the free weights, tossing him a resistance band.

David frowned. "What's this for? Strangling myself after this workout?"

Jake chuckled. "Nah, that's for later. Right now, it's for warming up."

David sighed and looped the band around his wrists, following Jake's lead as they worked through shoulder mobility drills. His muscles protested every movement, but after a few minutes, the stiffness started to fade.

"Alright," Jake said, cracking his knuckles. "Today, we're upping the intensity."

David groaned. "Of course we are."

Jake grabbed a pair of dumbbells. "We're doing a circuit. No long breaks, no slacking."

David gave him a deadpan look. "You *do* realize I still feel like I got run over by a truck, right?"

Jake smirked. "Perfect. Then let's hit round one."

The first circuit wasn't *that* bad.

The second circuit was worse.

By the third round, David was convinced his soul was trying to escape his body.

He dropped onto the bench, gasping for breath. "Jake—buddy—pal—why do you *hate* me?"

Jake laughed, barely winded. "I *like* you, Carter. That's why I'm making you better."

David groaned, wiping sweat from his forehead. His muscles were shaking, his breath uneven.

This was his breaking point.

He could feel it—the moment when he had to decide if he was going to quit or push through.

Jake knelt beside him, serious now. "Look, I know this sucks. But this right here? This is where most people give up. The second it gets too hard, they walk away. But that's not you. Not this time."

David closed his eyes, inhaling deeply.

He *wanted* to stop.

But he *needed* to keep going.

He clenched his fists, exhaled, and stood back up.

"Alright," he said, shaking out his arms. "One more round."

Jake grinned. "That's what I'm talking about."

David grabbed the weights, gritting his teeth.

This wasn't about finishing the workout.

This was about proving to himself that he *could*.

MARK FLORY

The Moment of Truth

David gripped the dumbbells, his muscles trembling. Sweat dripped down his forehead, his breaths came in short gasps, and every fiber of his being screamed for him to quit.

But he wasn't going to.

Not this time.

"Alright," Jake said, standing beside him. "Last set. Give me everything you've got."

David exhaled sharply. He planted his feet, rolled his shoulders, and hoisted the weights.

The first rep was shaky. His arms burned. His chest tightened.

The second rep felt even heavier, but he pushed through.

By the third rep, his body was threatening to give out.

Jake's voice cut through the exhaustion. "Don't stop. Fight through it."

David gritted his teeth.

One more.

His arms shook as he pushed the dumbbells up for the fourth rep. His breath hitched, and for a moment, he thought he might drop them.

But he didn't.

With a guttural groan, he forced the last rep up and slammed the weights onto the floor.

He collapsed onto the bench, completely spent. His entire body felt like it had been wrung out.

Jake clapped him on the shoulder. "That—right there—is how you break through."

David sucked in a breath, wiping sweat from his eyes.

It had been brutal. Painful.

But deep down, past the exhaustion, he felt something else. Something he hadn't felt in a long time.

Pride.

He looked up at Jake, shaking his head. "You really enjoy torturing me, huh?"

Jake grinned. "Nah. I enjoy watching people realize they're capable of more than they thought."

David chuckled weakly. "So... does this mean I survived?"

Jake smirked. "For today."

David exhaled, standing up slowly. His legs wobbled, his arms felt like jelly, but he didn't care.

He had shown up. He had done the work.

And tomorrow, he'd do it again.

Because for the first time in years, he *wasn't* breaking down.

He was breaking *through*.

CHAPTER 6

THE TRANSFORMATION BEGINS

Small Wins, Big Changes

David shuffled into his house, his body aching in ways he hadn't thought possible. His muscles were tight, his arms felt like dead weight, and he was convinced he'd need a forklift to get himself onto the couch.

Lisa glanced up from her laptop, smirking. "Well, you're still alive."

David groaned, dropping onto the couch with a dramatic sigh. "Barely."

She laughed. "Rough workout?"

David exhaled. "Jake tried to kill me again. Pretty sure I saw my life flash before my eyes."

Lisa leaned forward. "But you finished it?"

David nodded, rubbing his sore arms. "Yeah. Somehow."

Lisa smiled. "That's progress."

David thought about that for a moment.

She was right.

Two weeks ago, he wouldn't have even made it to the gym. A week ago, he would have made excuses to skip. And today?

He had shown up. Pushed through.

And despite the pain, he felt... good.

Lisa closed her laptop and slid onto the couch next to him. "I can already see the difference, you know."

David raised an eyebrow. "I haven't lost twenty pounds overnight, if that's what you mean."

Lisa rolled her eyes. "I mean in *you*. Your energy. The way you carry yourself. You seem... different."

David exhaled, staring at the ceiling. "Yeah. I feel different."

Not *fixed*. Not *perfect*.

But different.

And maybe—just maybe—that was the first step toward becoming the man he wanted to be.

When the Mirror Shows Progress

The next morning, David woke up before his alarm.

That alone was strange.

He lay there for a moment, blinking at the ceiling, waiting for the usual exhaustion to hit—the heavy weight of grogginess, the mental fog that kept him in bed for an extra twenty minutes.

But it didn't come.

Instead, his body *wanted* to move.

He stretched his arms overhead, expecting pain to shoot through his muscles. It was still there, but it wasn't the same brutal soreness as before. It was a dull ache, the kind that felt *earned.*

A small sign of progress.

He swung his legs over the bed and stood up, walking to the bathroom. As he flipped on the light, his eyes landed on the mirror.

And then he *really* looked at himself.

He wasn't ripped. He wasn't suddenly lean and muscular.

But there were *changes.*

His face looked less puffy. His shoulders had a little more definition. Even his posture was different—less slouched, more solid.

He turned slightly, running a hand over his stomach. It wasn't gone, but it wasn't *as bad* as before.

For the first time in years, the man staring back at him didn't look... lost.

He looked like someone who was fighting.

Lisa's voice drifted from behind him. "Checking yourself out?"

David smirked, turning. "Just making sure I'm still me."

She walked up beside him, resting a hand on his arm. "You are. Just a better version."

David exhaled.

It wasn't just about weight loss. It wasn't just about muscle.

It was about feeling *alive* again.

And for the first time in a long time... he did.

A New Routine

David laced up his sneakers, his body still adjusting to this new version of himself—the one who woke up early without hitting snooze, the one who didn't dread workouts but expected them.

Lisa watched from the kitchen, sipping her coffee. "Heading to the gym?"

David nodded, grabbing his water bottle. "Yeah. Gotta keep the streak going."

Lisa smirked. "Who are you, and what have you done with my husband?"

David chuckled. "No idea. But I think I like this guy better."

Lisa walked over and kissed his cheek. "So do I."

That gave him a boost.

He climbed into his car and drove to the gym, the same place that had once felt intimidating, like a place where other people belonged—not him.

Now, it was different.

Walking through the doors didn't feel like a chore. It felt like a choice.

Jake was already inside, warming up. He nodded when he saw David. "Look who's turning into a regular."

David smirked. "Don't get used to it."

Jake grinned. "Too late."

They started their warm-up, and David felt something shift.

The weights weren't lighter, but they felt manageable. The treadmill still sucked, but it didn't feel like torture.

His body was adapting.

His mind was changing.

Jake clapped him on the back between sets. "You noticing it yet?"

David wiped sweat from his forehead. "Yeah."

Jake nodded. "That's the thing about transformation—it sneaks up on you."

David exhaled.

He had spent years feeling stuck, thinking change was impossible.

But now?

Now he was becoming something new.

And he wasn't stopping anytime soon.

The First Real Test

David's body still ached, but it was a *good* ache. The kind that reminded him he was doing something right.

He and Jake moved through the gym, finishing their last round of weights. David dropped the dumbbells with a relieved sigh, rolling his shoulders.

"That's it?" he asked.

Jake smirked. "For today."

David shook his head. "You say that like it wasn't brutal."

Jake chuckled. "It *was* brutal. But you're handling it."

David grabbed his water bottle and took a long sip. He was still adjusting to the fact that he *was* handling it.

Just a couple of weeks ago, he had been struggling through every workout, barely surviving. Now, he was keeping up.

Jake wiped his hands on a towel. "Alright, Carter. I've got a challenge for you."

David narrowed his eyes. "Oh no. That sounds suspicious."

Jake grinned. "Relax. It's nothing crazy. I just want you to go one week—*one full week*—without breaking your nutrition plan. No cheats. No excuses."

David's stomach twisted.

The gym? He was getting used to that.

The food? That was still *hard*.

Jake must have seen his hesitation. "Look, man. You've been doing good. But this is where most people slip. They work out, they think that's enough, and they start cutting corners with food."

David exhaled. "I hear a 'but' coming."

Jake nodded. "*But* real results happen in the kitchen. And you know that."

David clenched his jaw. "No cheats. No excuses."

Jake nodded. "One week. Think you can do it?"

David thought about it. The happy hours, the late-night cravings, the habits that had ruled his life for years.

Then he thought about how far he'd come.

How much he *wanted* this.

He extended his hand. "One week. No cheats."

Jake shook it, grinning. "That's what I like to hear."

David grabbed his gym bag and headed toward the exit.

The workouts had been tough. The soreness had been brutal.

But this?

This might be the hardest test yet.

MARK FLORY

The Food Battle

David sat at the kitchen table, staring at his plate like it was his worst enemy.

Grilled chicken. Steamed broccoli. A small serving of quinoa.

Healthy. Clean. Exactly what he was *supposed* to eat.

And yet, all he could think about was the pizza Lisa had ordered for herself.

The smell filled the kitchen, warm and inviting, the melted cheese stretching as she pulled apart a slice. She caught him watching and smirked.

"You sure you don't want a bite?" she teased.

David exhaled, gripping his fork. "I hate you right now."

Lisa laughed. "Hey, *you* made this no-cheat deal with Jake."

David groaned, forcing himself to take a bite of his chicken. It was *fine*. It tasted good. But it wasn't pizza.

Lisa took another bite, chewing dramatically. "Mmm. So good."

David shot her a look. "You're enjoying this way too much."

She grinned. "A little."

He exhaled, looking back at his plate.

This was it. The real test.

It wasn't about *one* meal. It was about breaking the cycle.

All his past failed attempts started the same way—one excuse, one moment of *just this once*.

Not this time.

He chewed his chicken, swallowing hard. "One week. No cheats."

Lisa raised an eyebrow. "You're really sticking to this?"

David nodded. "Yeah."

Lisa set her pizza down, studying him. "You know... I think this is the most serious I've ever seen you about something like this."

David smirked. "It's because I usually quit before it gets real."

Lisa leaned forward. "And this time?"

David clenched his jaw. "This time, I finish."

Lisa smiled. "I like that."

David took another bite, pushing past the craving, past the temptation.

The old version of him would have caved.

But that guy?

He was gone.

CHAPTER 7

THE DISCIPLINE GAP

When Willpower is Tested

B y day three of his no-cheat challenge, David was feeling *good.*

His body felt lighter. His energy levels were steadier. The usual afternoon crashes weren't hitting as hard.

It was working.

But then—life decided to test him.

It started at work.

"Carter!" Mike called across the office, waving a donut in the air. "Come on, man. You *know* you want one."

David glanced at the breakroom table, which was covered in a dozen fresh, glazed temptations.

His stomach tightened.

Mike smirked, holding one out. "What's one little donut?"

David took a slow breath.

This was *exactly* the kind of moment that had derailed him in the past.

One slip.

One "just this once."

But he had come too far for that.

He shook his head. "Nah, man. I'm good."

Mike frowned. "Seriously?"

David nodded. "Seriously."

Mike let out a dramatic sigh. "Damn. New Carter is boring."

David smirked. "New Carter is focused."

Mike took a bite of his donut. "Your loss."

David turned back to his desk, exhaling.

One battle won.

But the day wasn't over yet.

That night, Lisa wanted to go out for dinner.

"Come on," she said, grabbing her coat. "You've been doing great. We'll find a place with healthy options."

David hesitated. "I don't know…"

Lisa raised an eyebrow. "You *do* realize you're allowed to eat outside of the house, right?"

David smirked. "Yeah, but restaurants are traps."

Lisa laughed. "So pick a place where you can win."

David exhaled. She had a point.

If he was going to make this lifestyle permanent, he had to learn how to navigate real-world situations.

Alright. Let's do this.

They ended up at a steakhouse.

Safe choice. Plenty of protein.

David scanned the menu, making sure he didn't fall into old habits. He ignored the burgers, skipped over the pasta, and zeroed in on the grilled salmon with roasted vegetables.

When the waiter arrived, Lisa ordered first. "I'll have the ribeye, medium, with mashed potatoes."

The waiter turned to David.

David took a breath. "Salmon. No butter. Extra veggies instead of rice."

The waiter nodded. "Good choice."

Lisa smirked. "Look at you, making solid choices out in the wild."

David chuckled. "Yeah, well, gotta prove to myself I can do it."

Lisa sipped her water. "You *are* doing it."

David leaned back in his chair, letting that sink in.

She was right.

For the first time in his life, he wasn't just *trying*.

He was *succeeding*.

The Mental Game

David sat across from Lisa, his fingers drumming lightly on the table as they waited for their meals.

The steakhouse buzzed with conversation and laughter, the smell of sizzling meat and buttered bread hanging thick in the air.

And then, the real test arrived.

The waiter set down a basket of warm, golden-brown dinner rolls.

Lisa smiled, grabbing one immediately, and slicing it open with a butter knife. The steam rose from the soft center as she spread butter over the top.

David swallowed hard.

He wasn't even a *bread guy*, but damn, that looked *good*.

Lisa caught him staring and grinned. "You sure you don't want one?"

David clenched his jaw. "I'm good."

Lisa tilted her head. "You *can* have one, you know."

David exhaled. "Yeah. But I won't."

Lisa studied him for a moment, then set her roll down. "You're really all in, huh?"

David nodded. "I have to be."

Lisa leaned forward. "I have to ask, though—why *now*? What's different this time?"

David thought about that.

He had tried before. Hell, he had *failed* before. Diets, workout plans, quick fixes. Nothing ever stuck.

But this? This felt... *real*.

He leaned back, exhaling. "Because I finally get it. It's not about motivation. It's not about waiting for some magical moment where everything feels easy."

Lisa raised an eyebrow. "So what's it about?"

David smirked. "Discipline. Showing up even when I don't feel like it."

Lisa nodded slowly. "That's the difference, then."

David took a sip of water. "Yeah. And I'm done making excuses."

Just then, their food arrived.

David looked down at his plate—grilled salmon, perfectly cooked, with bright, roasted vegetables.

This wasn't punishment.

This was fuel.

And for the first time in his life, he felt *in control*.

Owning the Choice

David took his first bite of salmon, letting the warm, flaky fish settle on his tongue. It tasted *good*. Clean. Light.

Not the same kind of satisfaction that came from a greasy burger or a loaded plate of pasta.

But *better*.

Because this was a choice—a deliberate one. And that made all the difference.

Lisa watched him as she cut into her steak. "So, be honest. Does it feel like you're missing out?"

David wiped his mouth with a napkin. "Honestly?" He shrugged. "Not really."

Lisa raised an eyebrow. "Seriously?"

David leaned back, thinking. "A few weeks ago? Yeah, I would have been fighting myself the whole time, convincing myself I *deserved* a cheat meal. But now? I don't feel like I'm being punished."

Lisa smirked. "That's called *growth*."

David chuckled. "More like *finally getting my act together*."

Lisa sipped her water, studying him. "So what's next?"

David frowned. "What do you mean?"

"I mean, you're eating better. You're working out. You've got momentum. Where's it leading?"

David sat with that question for a second.

At first, it had just been about survival—getting his body back under control, proving to himself that he *could* change.

But now?

Now, he wanted *more*.

He wanted to see how far he could push himself. How strong he could get. How much energy he could build.

He wanted to feel *better than ever*.

David set his fork down. "I don't know exactly. But I do know one thing."

Lisa leaned in. "What's that?"

David smirked. "I'm not stopping."

Lisa smiled. "Good. Because I kind of like this version of you."

David exhaled, taking another bite.

For the first time in a long time, he wasn't wondering *if* he could stick to something.

He *knew* he could.

Because this wasn't about losing weight.

It wasn't about looking better.

It was about proving to himself that he was *in control* of his life again.

And nothing—*nothing*—was going to take that from him.

When No One's Watching

David walked into the house feeling lighter—not physically, but *mentally*.

The dinner out had been a test, and he had passed. He had made the right choices, not out of guilt or obligation, but because he *wanted* to.

That was new.

Lisa set her purse on the counter and stretched. "I'm heading to bed. You coming?"

David glanced at the clock—9:45 PM. Normally, this was the time when he'd crash on the couch, watch TV, or maybe snack on something unhealthy.

But tonight, something tugged at him.

"Not yet," he said. "I think I'm gonna go for a walk."

Lisa paused, studying him. "A walk?"

David shrugged. "Yeah. Just a short one. Clear my head."

Lisa smiled. "Look at you. Who *is* this guy?"

David smirked. "No idea. But I think I like him."

Lisa kissed his cheek. "I do too."

The night air was crisp as David stepped outside.

The neighborhood was quiet, the streetlights casting long shadows along the sidewalk.

He started walking, hands in his pockets, letting his mind wander.

This was different from his usual routine. Normally, if he wasn't at the gym, he wasn't doing *anything*.

But tonight, his body *wanted* to move.

It wasn't about burning calories. It wasn't about checking off a box.

It was just about *being better*.

He passed by houses with their lights still on, glimpses of families watching TV, couples laughing over dinner.

And for the first time in a long time, he didn't feel like he was missing out.

He was *building* something.
Not just muscle. Not just discipline.
A *new* version of himself.
One who didn't make excuses. One who didn't quit.
One who did the work, even when no one was watching.

David stopped at the corner, taking a deep breath, feeling the cool air fill his lungs.

Then he turned around and walked home.
Tomorrow would be another challenge.
But for the first time, he wasn't afraid of it.
He was *ready*.

The Late-Night Craving

David stepped back into the house, his body relaxed from the walk, his mind clear.

It was late. Lisa was already asleep. The house was quiet.
And then—it hit him.
The craving.

Like a shadow creeping in from the corners of his mind, it whispered the old familiar temptation.

Just a little snack.

His stomach wasn't even *hungry*, but the habit was still there. The one that had led to years of mindless eating.

He walked into the kitchen, staring at the fridge.

He knew what was inside. Leftovers. Snacks. Things that *wouldn't* technically break his no-cheat week—but would feed the wrong habit.

He clenched his jaw.

This was the real fight.
Not the gym. Not the treadmill. Not the weights. *This*.
Standing here, alone, with no one watching.
If he caved, no one would know. No one would judge him.
But *he* would know.
He exhaled and opened the fridge.
His eyes landed on a protein shake. He grabbed it, shut the door, and leaned against the counter, sipping slowly.
It wasn't about *what* he ate. It was about *why*.
And tonight, he had made the right call.
Because this wasn't about willpower.
It was about *control*. And for the first time in a long time, *he* was in control.
David exhaled, set the empty bottle in the sink, and turned off the kitchen light.
Tomorrow was another day. And he was ready for it.

CHAPTER 8

BREAKING THE PLATEAU

The Comfort Trap

David stood in front of the mirror, shirtless, inspecting himself.

He wasn't where he wanted to be yet—but damn, he was different.

His face looked leaner. His arms had definition. His stomach, while not flat, wasn't spilling over his waistband anymore.

Progress.

But something felt... *stuck*.

He was still eating clean. Still showing up to the gym. Still doing *everything right*.

And yet, the changes were slowing down.

Lisa walked past the bathroom, stopping when she saw him. "Checking yourself out again?"

David smirked. "Just making sure I'm still me."

Lisa leaned against the door frame. "You look great."

David exhaled. "I feel great. But... I don't know. I think I've hit a wall."

Lisa frowned. "What do you mean?"

David rubbed his jaw. "The first few weeks, I could *see* the difference every few days. Now? Feels like I'm just coasting."

Lisa tilted her head. "So what's the plan?"

David sighed. "I have no idea."

Lisa smiled. "I bet Jake does."

David chuckled. "Yeah. And I bet I'm *not* gonna like it."

Lisa winked. "Probably not."

David grabbed his phone, already dreading what was coming.

David: *"Alright, coach. I think I hit a plateau."*

Jake's reply came almost instantly.

Jake: *"Good. That means we get to level up."*

David exhaled.

He had a *very* bad feeling about this.

The Next Level

David arrived at the gym, already regretting texting Jake.

He spotted his friend near the squat racks, adjusting weights with an all-too-excited grin. That was never a good sign.

David groaned. "I knew I was going to hate this."

HEALING ME NOW

Jake smirked. "You said you hit a plateau, right?"

David crossed his arms. "Yeah... which I *immediately* regretted telling you."

Jake laughed. "Good. That means you're about to grow."

David sighed. "So what's the deal? More weight? More reps?"

Jake shook his head. "Nope. *Intensity.* We're changing the way you train."

David frowned. "What does that even mean?"

Jake grabbed a kettlebell and handed it to him. "It means we're adding supersets, high-intensity intervals, and *absolutely no* long breaks."

David stared at the kettlebell. "This sounds awful."

Jake grinned. "It will be."

David exhaled, rolling his shoulders. "Alright. Let's do this."

The first circuit was brutal.

Squats into kettlebell swings. Push-ups straight into shoulder presses.

By the third round, David's lungs were on fire. Sweat dripped from his face, his arms felt like rubber, and his heart pounded against his ribs.

He bent over, gasping. "This... is *insane.*"

Jake grinned. "It's exactly what you need."

David wiped his face, shaking his head. "What happened to normal workouts?"

Jake chuckled. "Normal workouts got you here. But *this*? This is what's going to take you to the next level."

David groaned, rolling his shoulders. "I hate that you're right."

Jake smirked. "You're gonna hate me more in five minutes."

David exhaled, standing up. "Fine. What's next?"

Jake's grin widened. "Sprints."

David's stomach dropped. "Oh, *come on.*"

Jake clapped him on the back. "No plateaus on my watch, Carter. Let's go."

David shook his head.

This was going to suck.

But if it got him *unstuck*?

He was all in.

The Sprint That Changed Everything

David stood at the edge of the track, hands on his hips, already drenched in sweat.

Sprints.

Why did it *have* to be sprints?

Jake stood beside him, completely at ease. "Alright, Carter. Here's the deal. Ten rounds. Thirty seconds all-out sprint, followed by a sixty-second walk."

David groaned. "You *do* realize my legs barely survived the last workout, right?"

Jake smirked. "And yet, here you are."

David sighed, rolling his shoulders. "Let's get this over with."

Jake nodded. "Alright. First round. Full effort. Go!"

David took off, pumping his arms, his legs driving forward.

At first, it wasn't *that* bad. The fresh air, the rhythm of his breath, the burn in his muscles—it felt *good.*

Then, at the twenty-second mark, his lungs caught fire.

His legs slowed, his breath came in ragged gasps, and by the time Jake yelled "Walk!" he was *barely* holding himself together.

David hunched over, hands on his knees. "Oh... my... God..."

Jake chuckled. "One down. Nine to go."

David groaned. "You're actually insane."

Jake smirked. "And you're actually doing it."

By the eighth round, David was *done.*

His legs felt like cement. His chest heaved. Sweat poured down his face.

His brain screamed at him to stop.

You've done enough.

No one would blame you if you quit now.

Jake jogged up beside him. "Two more, Carter."

David clenched his fists.

He could quit.

Or—

He could finish.

He looked up at Jake. "Alright. Let's go."

Jake grinned. "That's the spirit."

David inhaled, gritted his teeth—

And sprinted.

The Final Sprint

David's legs burned like they were filled with molten lead. His lungs screamed for mercy. Every fiber of his body told him to stop.

But he *didn't.*

Because this was the moment that mattered.

Not the first sprint. Not the easy rounds.

This one.

The one where everything in him wanted to quit—but he *chose* not to.

Jake ran beside him, keeping pace, his voice cutting through the exhaustion. "Come on, Carter! Empty the tank!"

David clenched his jaw and pushed harder, his arms pumping, his legs driving forward.

Twenty seconds left.

The world blurred around him. His breath came in short, sharp bursts.

Fifteen seconds.

His muscles screamed, his body begged for a break.

Ten seconds.

He pushed *past* the pain.

Five seconds.

Jake yelled, "Finish strong!"

David gritted his teeth, gave everything he had left—

And crossed the line.

He slowed to a stop, hands on his knees, gasping for air. His heart pounded like a war drum in his chest. Sweat poured from his face.

But he had done it.

All ten rounds.

No quitting. No excuses.

Jake clapped him on the back, grinning. "That, my friend, is *how* you break a plateau."

David shook his head, still trying to catch his breath. "I... hate... you."

Jake laughed. "You'll thank me tomorrow."

David groaned, dropping onto the grass. "I doubt that."

Jake smirked. "No, you *will*. Because this, this is where it all changes."

David exhaled, staring up at the sky.

Jake was right.

He had felt stuck, like his progress was stalling. But now?

Now, he knew he had *so much more* to give.

And this wasn't just about breaking a plateau.

This was about breaking *limits*.

The Shift in Mindset

David lay on the grass, his chest rising and falling in deep, uneven breaths. His body was spent. Completely drained.

And yet... he felt *alive*.

Jake sat down next to him, tossing him a bottle of water. "You did good today."

David grabbed the bottle, twisting off the cap with shaky hands. "Felt like hell."

Jake chuckled. "That's because it *was* hell. But you didn't stop."

David took a long sip of water, wiping sweat from his face. "Didn't think I had it in me."

Jake smirked. "That's the thing, Carter. Most people don't know what they're capable of. They stop when it gets *hard*, thinking that's their limit."

David exhaled. "And it's not?"

Jake shook his head. "Nope. Your real limit is *way* past what your brain tells you."

David thought about that.

All his life, he had given up when things got tough. When the soreness hit. When the cravings got bad. When life threw distractions his way.

But today?

He had kept going.

Not because it was easy. Not because it felt good.

But because he *chose* to.

Jake leaned back on his elbows. "This is the shift, man. You're not just working out anymore. You're not just dieting. You're *reprogramming* yourself."

David nodded slowly. "Yeah... I think I get it now."

Jake smiled. "Good. Because from here on out, the only way is forward."

David sat up, rolling his sore shoulders. His body ached, but his mind felt *stronger* than ever.

He wasn't *trying* anymore.

He *was* changing.

And this time?

There was no going back.

CHAPTER 9

BECOMING THE MAN HE WAS MEANT TO BE

A New Standard

David woke up the next morning expecting to feel wrecked. But instead of the deep, crushing soreness that had haunted him after his first workouts, he felt... *strong*.

Sure, his legs were stiff, and his arms still ached, but it wasn't the kind of pain that made him want to stay in bed.

It was the kind of pain that *proved* he was getting better.

He sat up, stretching, rolling his shoulders.

Lisa stirred beside him, groggy. "You're up early."

David smirked. "So are you."

She yawned. "Only because you moved."

David chuckled, swinging his legs over the side of the bed. "I think my body's just getting used to it."

Lisa blinked at him. "Used to what?"

David stood, rolling out his shoulders. "The work."

Lisa watched him for a moment. Then she smiled. "I like this version of you."

David turned to her, stretching his arms. "Yeah... me too."

At the gym, Jake was already there, as usual, finishing a warm-up set.

David approached, feeling lighter than usual.

Jake grinned. "Look at you. Walking in here like you *want* to be here."

David smirked. "Shocking, I know."

Jake set down his weights. "Let me guess. The plateau's not a problem anymore?"

David shook his head. "Nope."

Jake nodded. "Good. Because that means we raise the standard again."

David exhaled, rolling his neck. "Of course we do."

Jake laughed. "Hey, that's what this is about, right? You don't just *get* better. You keep getting better."

David cracked his knuckles.

A few months ago, he would've dreaded those words.

But now?

Now, he welcomed them.

Because he wasn't just working out.

He was becoming *the man he was meant to be.*

The Strength Test

David stood in front of the squat rack, rolling his shoulders. The last time he had done this, it had nearly destroyed him.

But today?

Today, he was *ready*.

Jake loaded the bar with more weight than David had ever lifted before. Not by much—but just enough to test him.

"Alright," Jake said, stepping back. "This is your moment, Carter."

David exhaled, stepping under the bar. The steel rested on his shoulders, heavier than he expected.

Jake's voice was steady. "Breathe. Core tight. Control the descent."

David took a slow breath, then lowered himself into the squat.

His legs shook slightly. His mind screamed, *too heavy, too much, too soon.*

But his body?

His body *knew* better.

He pushed up.

The weight moved. Slowly at first—then stronger, steadier.

Before he knew it, he was standing tall again, the bar locked in place.

Jake grinned. "Hell yeah."

David racked the bar and stepped back, his heart pounding.

He had done it.

No fear. No hesitation.

Just *strength*.

Jake clapped him on the back. "Told you. You're stronger than you think."

David wiped sweat from his forehead, grinning. "Yeah... I think I finally believe it."

Jake smirked. "Good. Because we're adding more next week."

David chuckled. "Of course we are."

This wasn't the finish line.

This was just the *beginning*.

The Mental Shift

David sat on a bench, still catching his breath. His legs felt like jelly, his arms hung heavy at his sides, but deep down—past the exhaustion—he felt something new.

Control.

Jake handed him a bottle of water. "How's it feel?"

David took a sip, letting the cold liquid cool his burning throat. He wiped the sweat from his forehead and smirked. "Feels like I can do more."

Jake grinned. "That's the difference, Carter. A month ago, you were just trying to *survive* the workouts. Now, you're chasing the next level."

David leaned forward, resting his elbows on his knees. "Yeah. And I don't think it's just about the gym anymore."

Jake raised an eyebrow. "What do you mean?"

David exhaled, staring at the floor. "For the longest time, I just... let life happen to me. Work, eating, bad habits—it all felt automatic, like I wasn't even *in control.*"

Jake nodded. "And now?"

David looked up, confidence settling into his voice. "Now I *am* in control."

Jake smiled. "That's the mindset shift, man. The moment when fitness isn't just about lifting weights—it's about how you *see* yourself. You're not the same guy who walked in here weeks ago."

David rolled his shoulders. "Yeah. I'm not."

He stood up, stretching his sore legs. He wasn't just chasing a number on the scale or a certain look in the mirror.

He was chasing *himself*.

The version of him that didn't make excuses.

The version of him that didn't quit.

The version of him that had been buried under years of doubt and bad decisions—but was finally breaking free.

Jake clapped him on the back. "Alright, Carter. You ready for the next challenge?"

David smirked. "Always."

This wasn't just a fitness journey anymore.

This was *who he was becoming.*

And he wasn't turning back.

MARK FLORY

The Unexpected Challenge

David walked out of the gym feeling invincible. His body was sore, but it was the *good* kind—the soreness that came from pushing limits and breaking barriers.

He had been stuck for so long, but now? Now, he was *moving forward.*

And then—life threw a curveball.

His phone buzzed. A message from his boss.

Boss: *"Carter, I need you in early tomorrow. We've got a problem."*

David frowned.

His mornings were sacred now. Gym first, work second. That was the rule he had built for himself.

He glanced at the time. It was already late. If he had to go in early, it meant one thing—he'd have to *skip* his workout.

He clenched his jaw.

Skipping wasn't an option.

Not anymore.

David took a deep breath and called his boss.

"Hey, boss," he said. "I'll be there early, but I need an hour before we start. I have a commitment."

There was a pause on the other end. "A commitment?"

David exhaled. "Yeah. My morning workout. It's non-negotiable."

His boss chuckled. "You're serious?"

David nodded. "Yeah. I'll come in early, but I need that hour first."

Silence.

Then, finally—

"Alright, Carter. I respect that. See you after your 'non-negotiable.'"

David smirked. "See you then."

He hung up, exhaling.

The old version of him would've dropped everything for work.

The new version?

He protected his priorities.

Because this wasn't *just* a fitness journey.

It was about *who he was becoming.*

And that man?

He didn't make excuses.

He made it happen.

Commitment Over Convenience

The next morning, David's alarm blared at 4:45 AM.

He groaned, rubbing his face. It was earlier than he was used to. Earlier than he *wanted.*

But he had made a commitment.

And if there was one thing he was learning, it was that discipline wasn't about doing things when they were convenient. It was about doing them *anyway.*

He got up, stretched his sore muscles, and pulled on his gym clothes.

Lisa stirred, squinting at him in the dark. "It's *so* early. You sure you don't want to skip today?"

David smirked. "Not an option."

Lisa smiled sleepily. "Proud of you."

David kissed her forehead and headed out the door.

The gym was nearly empty when he arrived.

Jake wasn't there—he didn't even *know* about this early session. This wasn't about meeting expectations or proving something to someone else.

This was about proving something to *himself.*

David warmed up, shaking off the early-morning sluggishness. The weights felt heavy, but he pushed through. Every rep, every movement reminded him why he was doing this.

By the time he finished his workout, the sun was just starting to rise.

He walked out of the gym feeling *different.*

Not just physically.

But *mentally.*

The old David would've hit snooze. Would've made an excuse.

The new David?

He *showed up.*

And that made all the difference.

As he got into his car and drove to work, he realized something:

This wasn't just about fitness anymore.

This was about *who he was choosing to be—every single day.*

And for the first time in a long time, he *liked* who that was.

CHAPTER 10

THE TURNING POINT

The Moment It Clicked

David walked into the office, his muscles still warm from the early workout.

For the first time in years, he *felt ahead*—like he had already won the day before it even started.

No rushing. No sluggish, half-asleep mornings.

Just clarity. Control.

Mike looked up from his desk and smirked. "Well, look who's all energized at the crack of dawn."

David chuckled, setting his coffee down. "Something like that."

Mike shook his head. "Dude, you used to drag yourself in here half-dead every morning. Now you're... *different.*"

David exhaled, leaning back in his chair. "Yeah. I guess I am."

Mike raised an eyebrow. "So what changed?"

David thought about that.

At first, it was just about getting *back* in shape. Losing weight. Fixing bad habits.

But somewhere along the way, it had become more than that.

It wasn't just about looking better.

It was about *being* better.

David shrugged. "I stopped negotiating with myself."

Mike frowned. "What does that mean?"

David smirked. "It means I don't give myself an out anymore. I don't wake up and ask, 'Do I feel like going to the gym?' I just *go*. I don't ask, 'Do I really need to eat healthy today?' I just *do it*."

Mike leaned back, considering that. "Huh. That's actually kinda badass."

David chuckled. "Took me long enough to figure it out."

Mike smirked. "Well, whatever you're doing, it's working. I might need to steal some of that motivation."

David shook his head. "It's not motivation, man. It's discipline."

Mike nodded slowly. "Yeah... I think I get that now."

David sipped his coffee, staring out the window.

It had taken him years to get to this point.

But now that he was here?

He *wasn't going back.*

Leading by Example

The workday passed in a blur. Meetings, emails, the usual office grind.

But something was *different*.

David felt sharper. More focused. The usual afternoon slump never came.

By the time lunch rolled around, he grabbed his prepped meal from the fridge—grilled chicken, roasted sweet potatoes, and a side of greens.

Mike walked by, holding a greasy burger in one hand and a soda in the other. He paused, eyeing David's meal. "You *actually* meal prep now?"

David smirked. "Yeah. Saves time. Saves bad decisions."

Mike shook his head. "Man, I don't know how you do it. I always tell myself I'll eat clean, but then…" He lifted his burger. "This happens."

David chuckled. "It's not about being perfect, Mike. It's about controlling what you *can* control."

Mike hesitated, then sat down. "Alright, tell me the truth. Do you ever miss it? The junk food? The beer? Just *eating whatever*?"

David thought about that.

Did he miss it?

Sure. Sometimes.

But what he *didn't* miss was the sluggishness. The bloating. The feeling of being stuck in his own body.

He shook his head. "Not really. Because I know how I feel *after* I eat clean. And that's worth more than any burger."

Mike studied him for a moment, then nodded. "Yeah. I respect that."

David smirked. "Besides, you don't have to quit everything. Just make better choices *most* of the time."

Mike chewed his lip. "Alright, Carter. I'll bite. What's one easy thing I can do *today* to get started?"

David grinned. "Swap that soda for water. Start small."

Mike exhaled. "Fine. But if I die from lack of sugar, it's on you."

David laughed, shaking his head.

He wasn't trying to preach. He wasn't trying to convert anyone.

But something was happening.

People were *noticing*.

And maybe—just maybe—his journey wasn't just changing him.

The Ripple Effect

David hadn't set out to inspire anyone.

He was just trying to fix himself.

But now, people were *watching*.

It wasn't just Mike. Others in the office had started asking him questions—little things at first.

"What protein powder do you use?"

"How do you meal prep without getting bored?"

"Dude, are you actually *enjoying* working out now?"

It was subtle, but he could feel it.

His discipline was creating a ripple effect.

And that?

That was something he never expected.

That evening, he was at home stretching when Lisa walked in with a curious expression.

"So, I ran into Sarah at the store today," she said, sitting down on the couch.

David raised an eyebrow. "Sarah from your office?"

Lisa nodded. "Yeah. She asked me what's been different with you lately. Said she could tell you were *changing*—not just physically, but the way you carry yourself."

David exhaled, leaning back. "Huh."

Lisa smirked. "You know what I told her?"

David shrugged. "What?"

Lisa smiled. "I told her you finally decided to *show up for yourself*."

David thought about that.

She was right.

For years, he had gone through the motions—at work, at home, even in his own mind. He had *existed*, but he hadn't *lived*.

Now?

Now he was *choosing* himself. Every day.

And that choice?

It was starting to change *everything*.

Owning the New Identity

David sat on the back patio, sipping a glass of water, watching the sun dip below the horizon.

Lisa had gone inside to finish up some work, and for the first time all day, he was alone with his thoughts.

He thought about Sarah's comment. About Mike ditching his soda. About the way people were starting to notice.

He wasn't just a guy *trying* to get healthy anymore.

He *was* that guy now.

And that realization hit him harder than any workout ever had.

His phone buzzed.

Jake: *"How's the body holding up?"*

David smirked and typed back.

David: *"Better than ever."*

Jake's response was quick.

Jake: *"Good. Because we're leveling up tomorrow."*

David chuckled.

Of course they were.

And for the first time, he wasn't nervous about what that meant.

He was *ready*.

Because this wasn't just a phase. This was *who he was now*.

No More Limits

David walked into the gym the next morning with a different energy.

For weeks, he had been *pushing* himself, breaking past old habits, learning discipline.

But today?

Today, he wasn't *pushing* himself.

He was *owning* this.

Jake spotted him from across the gym, grinning. "Look at you, walking in like you belong here."

David smirked. "Because I do."

Jake laughed, tossing him a resistance band. "Alright, big man. Time to test some limits."

David rolled his shoulders. "I don't have limits anymore."

Jake raised an eyebrow. "That so?"

David nodded. "Yeah. Because limits are just excuses you haven't challenged yet."

Jake grinned. "I like that. Now let's put it to the test."

The workout was brutal. Heavier weights. Faster transitions. Less rest.

The kind of session that would've *broken* him a month ago.

But today?

He powered through.

Every rep. Every set.

No hesitation.

No doubt.

Just work.

By the end, he was drenched in sweat, his heart pounding—but he wasn't *wrecked*.

He was *strong*.

Jake clapped him on the back. "Damn, Carter. You're a different animal now."

David wiped his face with a towel, breathing deeply. "Nah. I'm just the guy I was always supposed to be."

Jake smirked. "That's dangerous."

David chuckled. "For my excuses? Yeah."

He grabbed his water bottle and headed toward the exit.

This wasn't just another workout.

This wasn't just another day.
This was *who he was now*.
And there was no going back.

CHAPTER 11

BUILDING THE FUTURE

The Next Step

David sat at his desk, staring at an open email draft.

It was from his boss—an invitation to lead a team project. A *big* one.

A few months ago, he wouldn't have even considered it. He would have convinced himself that he wasn't ready, that someone else was better suited for the challenge.

But now?

Now, he *knew* better.

His transformation wasn't just about the gym. It was about the way he approached *everything*—work, relationships, and most of all, himself.

No more hesitation.

No more second-guessing.

He clicked **Reply** and typed:

"I'm in. Let's get started."

That evening, he met Jake at the gym.

Jake leaned against the squat rack, smirking. "You're looking extra confident today."

David chuckled, rolling his shoulders. "I finally figured something out."

Jake raised an eyebrow. "Oh yeah? What's that?"

David picked up a weight, testing the grip. "All this time, I was waiting to *feel* ready. But being ready isn't a feeling. It's a decision."

Jake grinned. "Now you're getting it."

David smirked. "Took me long enough."

Jake clapped his hands together. "Alright then. Since you're all about *decisions* now, here's one—heavy squats or sled pushes?"

David cracked his neck.

"Both."

Jake laughed. "I was hoping you'd say that."

David stepped toward the rack, gripping the bar with steady hands.

He wasn't the same man who started this journey.

And he never would be again.

Because now?

He was *building the future he deserved.*

Strength Beyond the Gym

David pressed the bar off the squat rack, feeling its weight settle onto his shoulders.

Heavy. But not impossible.

He inhaled, steadied his stance, and lowered himself. His legs burned, but he *owned* the movement—controlled, strong, unshaken.

He pushed up, locking out the rep.

Jake grinned. "Easy."

David smirked. "Not easy. Just *earned*."

He set the bar back onto the rack, shaking out his legs.

Jake tossed him a towel. "You're getting stronger, Carter."

David wiped the sweat from his face. "Yeah, and not just here."

Jake tilted his head. "Oh?"

David took a deep breath. "For years, I let myself coast. Physically, mentally, at work... everywhere. I'd show up, do what I had to, but I wasn't really *trying*. Wasn't really *invested*."

Jake nodded. "And now?"

David exhaled, clenching his fists. "Now, I don't accept *half-assed* anymore. Not in the gym. Not in life."

Jake smirked. "So, what's next?"

David grabbed his water bottle, rolling his shoulders.

"I stop *building back*—and start *building forward*."

Jake chuckled. "Damn right."

They moved to the sled track.

Jake loaded the plates. "Alright. No limits, right?"

David grinned.

"No limits."

And as he gripped the sled and drove forward, pushing with everything he had—

He knew there was no going back.

Not now.

Not ever.

The Shift No One Expected

David sat at his desk, rolling his shoulders as he skimmed through emails.

A few months ago, this was the part of his day that drained him. Endless meetings, long hours, the feeling that he was just *getting through* the day instead of actually *living* it.

But now?

Now, everything felt *different*.

He was more focused. More efficient.

More *present*.

Mike strolled over, sipping a black coffee. "Alright, Carter. Spill it."

David raised an eyebrow. "Spill what?"

Mike gestured at him. "You. The new-and-improved, early-rising, weight-lifting, disciplined version of Carter. How do I get *that*?"

David smirked, leaning back. "You really wanna know?"

Mike nodded. "Yeah, man. Because whatever switch flipped for you? I need that."

David exhaled. "It's simple, but not easy."

Mike crossed his arms. "I'm listening."

HEALING ME NOW

David tapped his desk. "Stop negotiating with yourself. That's it."

Mike frowned. "What does that mean?"

David leaned forward. "It means you don't wait to *feel* like doing something. You just *do it.* You don't wake up and decide if today's a workout day. Every day *is* a workout day. You don't debate whether you should eat better. You just *do.*"

Mike let that sit for a moment.

Then he chuckled. "Damn. No wonder you're different."

David smirked. "You in?"

Mike sighed, rubbing his face. "Hell... I guess I *have* been coasting."

David grinned. "Then stop."

Mike shook his head, laughing. "You make it sound easy."

David's smirk faded. "It's not. But it's worth it."

Mike studied him for a moment, then nodded. "Alright. No more half-assed. I'm in."

David leaned back, satisfied.

This wasn't just about *his* future anymore.

It was about something *bigger.*

And that? That was just the beginning.

The First Recruit

David didn't expect to become a leader.
But here he was.

Mike had always been the guy cracking jokes, the guy who lived for happy hours and weekend binge sessions.

Now?

Now, he was asking *how to change*.

And David wasn't about to let him down.

The next morning, Mike met him at the gym.

He looked *rough*—hair still messy, dark circles under his eyes, and a very obvious, *what the hell am I doing here?* expression.

David smirked. "You look thrilled."

Mike groaned. "Dude, it's *five-thirty in the morning*. I hate everything."

David chuckled. "Yeah. You'll get over it."

Mike sighed. "Alright. Where do we start?"

David tossed him a resistance band. "With *humility*."

Mike frowned. "Huh?"

David crossed his arms. "You're not the guy you were in college. You're not as strong as you used to be. That's fine. But if you wanna do this right, you've gotta let go of the ego."

Mike chewed his lip, then nodded. "Fair."

David grinned. "Good. Now, warm up. We've got work to do."

The session was brutal.

Not because it was anything extreme—but because Mike wasn't *ready* for this.

By the second set of squats, he was drenched in sweat. By the third, he looked like he might throw up.

"You *do this* every day?" Mike gasped, hands on his knees.

David chuckled. "Yeah. And so will you."

Mike groaned. "This was a mistake."

David smirked. "Nah. The mistake was waiting this long to start."

Mike exhaled. "Damn. That's deep."

David tossed him a towel. "Yeah, well, get used to it. We're just getting started."

Mike took a long breath. "Alright. See you tomorrow?"
David grinned.
"You *know* it."

The Responsibility of Growth

David watched as Mike collapsed onto a nearby bench, gulping down water like a man who had just survived a desert trek.

"You're not dead," David said, smirking. "So that's a win."

Mike groaned. "I *feel* dead."

David chuckled, tossing him a protein bar. "Eat. You'll feel human again in about ten minutes."

Mike unwrapped it, shaking his head. "I don't know how you do this, man. The discipline, the early mornings, the no-crap diet..."

David exhaled, leaning against the wall. "Because I stopped making excuses."

Mike chewed, nodding slowly. "Yeah... I can see that." He swallowed and looked up. "I think that's what scares me the most."

David raised an eyebrow. "What does?"

Mike sighed. "The fact that if I *don't* change, it's *my fault*."

David let that sink in.

It was the same realization he had come to months ago—the moment he understood that *no one* was coming to save him.

That *he* was the problem.

And *he* was the solution.

David sat beside him. "Look, man. It's not about being perfect. It's about owning your choices."

Mike wiped sweat from his face. "No more hiding behind bad habits?"

David nodded. "No more pretending it's out of your control."

Mike exhaled. "Alright. I'm in."

David grinned. "Then get used to the grind, brother. Because this?" He gestured around the gym. "This is your new normal."

Mike groaned but smiled. "Guess I better survive, then."

David clapped him on the back. "Damn right."

Because this wasn't just about *his* journey anymore.

Now, he had people counting on him.

And that?

That was a responsibility he was ready for.

CHAPTER 12

LEADING THE WAY

Setting the Standard

D avid walked into the office the next morning, feeling the kind of energy he used to *wish* for.

No coffee-fueled struggle to wake up. No sluggish brain fog. Just clarity. Strength.

And the best part?

He wasn't the only one anymore.

Mike trailed behind him, still rubbing his sore arms. "Dude, I swear, my body is shutting down."

David smirked. "That's just your muscles waking up."

Mike groaned. "Tell them to go back to sleep."

David laughed, grabbing his meal-prepped lunch from the breakroom fridge. "You sore?"

Mike sighed. "Like hell."

David sat down. "Good. That means you're doing it right."

Mike collapsed into the chair across from him, stretching his arms. "Man, I gotta be honest. I didn't think I'd come back today."

David raised an eyebrow. "And yet, here you are."

Mike sighed. "Yeah. Because if *you* can do it, so can I."

David paused, letting that settle.

People were *watching* him.

Not because he was forcing them. Not because he was preaching about fitness or discipline.

But because he was *living* it.

And that?

That was leadership.

David leaned forward. "Then let's make a deal."

Mike narrowed his eyes. "Oh boy. Here we go."

David smirked. "One month. No quitting. No excuses. We show up, we put in the work, and we don't let the soreness win."

Mike exhaled. "One *month?*"

David nodded. "Yeah. Because if you can do it for a month, you can do it for life."

Mike drummed his fingers on the table, then extended his hand. "Alright, Carter. One month."

David shook it. "No turning back."

Mike sighed. "God help me."

David chuckled.

This wasn't just about fitness anymore.

This was about *leading by example.*

And he was ready.

The Test of Commitment

One week into their deal, Mike was *struggling*.
David could see it in the way he moved—slower, more hesitant, like every muscle in his body was screaming at him to quit.
And honestly?
That's what David expected.
Because this was the part where most people *gave up*.
The soreness, the mental fatigue, the old habits creeping back in.
The real test wasn't about showing up on *day one*.
It was about showing up on *day ten, twenty, thirty...* when the excitement wore off and the grind became *real*.
Mike leaned against the squat rack, shaking his head. "Man, I don't know if I can do this."
David crossed his arms. "What part?"
Mike sighed. "All of it. The waking up early, the meal prepping, the workouts..." He exhaled, rubbing his face. "I don't know how you do this every damn day."
David smirked. "I don't *do* it every day. I *am* it every day."
Mike frowned. "What's the difference?"
David leaned in. "The difference is that I don't *decide* every morning whether or not I'm going to work out. It's just *what I do*. No debate. No question."
Mike looked at him, something shifting behind his eyes.

David continued. "The moment you stop giving yourself a way out? That's the moment everything changes."

Mike nodded slowly. "So no more negotiating with myself?"

David grinned. "Exactly."

Mike took a deep breath, then nodded. "Alright. Let's finish this workout."

David clapped him on the back. "Now you're getting it."

Because this wasn't just about fitness.

This was about *becoming the kind of man who doesn't quit.*

And Mike?

He was *starting* to get it.

No More Halfway

By the end of the session, Mike was *wrecked.*

He sat on the floor, drenched in sweat, shaking his head. "I swear, Carter, you're trying to kill me."

David chuckled, tossing him a towel. "Nah, man. Just trying to kill the version of you that quits."

Mike groaned, wiping his face. "Well, he's *definitely* dying."

David smirked. "Good. Because that guy? He's the only thing standing between you and who you're supposed to be."

Mike exhaled, staring up at the ceiling. "Man... I don't know if I have that *next level* in me."

David sat down beside him. "That's what I used to think, too."

Mike glanced at him. "And?"

David leaned forward, elbows on his knees. "And then I stopped waiting to *feel* ready. I just *did the work.*"

Mike nodded slowly.

David continued. "You're at the hardest part right now. The place where most people *halfway commit*—just enough to feel like they're trying, but not enough to actually *change*."

Mike sighed. "Yeah... I don't wanna be that guy."

David smirked. "Then don't be."

Mike clenched his jaw, then stood up, rolling out his shoulders.

"Alright," he said. "No more halfway."

David grinned. "Now you're speaking my language."

Mike nodded. "Tomorrow. Same time?"

David extended his hand. "Every damn day."

Mike shook it.

No turning back now.

Pushing Through the Wall

The next morning, David was already warming up when Mike walked into the gym.

Mike looked exhausted—his movements slower, his eyes still heavy with sleep.

David raised an eyebrow. "Rough morning?"

Mike groaned. "Didn't sleep great. Almost skipped."

David smirked. "But you didn't."

Mike sighed. "Nope. Because I knew you'd never let me hear the end of it."

David chuckled, tossing him a resistance band. "Damn right. Now let's get to work."

The workout started slow, but David could tell Mike was struggling.

Every set looked heavier. Every movement was a little sloppier.

By the halfway point, Mike dropped onto the bench, breathing hard. "Man, I *don't have it* today."

David crossed his arms. "You do. You just don't *feel* like you do."

Mike wiped sweat from his forehead. "What's the difference?"

David leaned in. "The difference is showing up anyway."

Mike sighed, rubbing his face. "Dude, I don't know if I can push through this."

David sat next to him. "You *can*. And you will. Because this is where the real change happens—not on the days when it's easy, but on the days when everything in you wants to quit."

Mike exhaled, staring at the floor. "Man, I hate you sometimes."

David smirked. "Good. That means I'm doing my job."

Mike chuckled weakly.

Then, slowly, he stood up.

"Alright," he said. "One set at a time."

David grinned. "That's the only way."

Because this wasn't just about today's workout.

This was about *who Mike was becoming.*

And David wasn't letting him quit on that.

The Breakthrough

Mike stood in front of the squat rack, breathing heavily. His legs burned, his mind screamed at him to quit, but something inside him refused to give in.

David stood beside him, arms crossed. "Last set. You got this."

Mike exhaled. "What if I fail?"

David smirked. "Then you rack the bar, reset, and do it again."

Mike clenched his jaw, nodding. He stepped under the bar, gripping it tight.

This was the moment.

Not just of today's workout—but of *everything*.

The past version of him would have walked away, found an excuse, let fatigue win.

But *not today.*

Mike took a deep breath, lowered into the squat—

And *pushed up.*

His legs shook, his core engaged, and for a second, he thought he might not make it.

Then, suddenly—he was standing tall, the bar locked in place.

David grinned. "Hell yeah."

Mike racked the bar and stumbled back, laughing breathlessly. "Holy crap. I did it."

David clapped him on the back. "Damn right you did."

Mike bent over, hands on his knees, still catching his breath. Then he looked up, a new kind of fire in his eyes. "I think I get it now."

David raised an eyebrow. "Get what?"

Mike stood up, rolling his shoulders. "This whole thing. The discipline. The grind. It's not about lifting weights."

David smirked. "Nope."

Mike exhaled. "It's about *who you become* in the process."

David nodded. "Now you're speaking my language."

Mike chuckled. "Man, if you told me a month ago that I'd be excited to come back tomorrow, I would've called you insane."

David grinned. "And yet, here you are."

Mike extended a hand. "Appreciate you, Carter."

David shook it firmly. "We're just getting started."

Because this wasn't just about fitness anymore.

This was about *leading by example*.

And now, Mike *was all in.*

CHAPTER 13

A NEW STANDARD

The Shift That Sticks

D avid woke up before his alarm again.
It was becoming a pattern now—his body waking up naturally, energized, ready to *move*. No grogginess, no dragging himself out of bed like he used to.

Just purpose.

Lisa stirred beside him, squinting as she watched him get up. "You know... I don't even set an alarm for you anymore. You're up before it every day."

David smirked, stretching. "I think my body's finally accepted this is just how life works now."

Lisa rolled onto her side, resting her head on her hand. "You've changed, you know. Not just physically."

David sat on the edge of the bed, rubbing his jaw. "Yeah... I feel it too."

Lisa studied him. "Do you ever think about how far you've come?"

David exhaled. He hadn't really *stopped* to reflect.

Months ago, he was the guy who lived for comfort—hitting snooze, skipping workouts, eating whatever felt easy. Now, he was *this* guy.

The one who showed up. The one who put in the work. The one who *kept going*.

And it wasn't just in the gym.

He was more focused at work. More patient at home. More *present* in his own life.

Lisa reached for his hand. "I know you don't need me to say it, but I'm proud of you."

David squeezed her fingers gently. "I think... I'm proud of me too."

Lisa smiled. "So what's next?"

David stood, stretching his arms. "Whatever the next challenge is."

Lisa raised an eyebrow. "And what if the challenge isn't in the gym?"

David grinned. "Doesn't matter. I'll show up for it anyway."

And deep down, he knew—this wasn't a phase.

This was *who he was now*.

The Challenge Outside the Gym

David walked into the office with his usual confidence, shoulders back, energy high.

He had started to love this feeling—not just physically strong, but mentally sharp. Focused. Ready.

But today, the air felt different.

His boss, Greg, stood near the conference room, arms crossed, face tight with stress. When he spotted David, he waved him over.

"Carter, got a minute?"

David nodded, following him inside.

Greg shut the door, exhaling. "We've got a problem."

David sat down. "What's up?"

Greg ran a hand through his graying hair. "That project you took on? The client is pushing back. They want revisions *yesterday*. And honestly, if we don't deliver fast, we could lose the account."

David leaned forward. "Alright. What do we need to do?"

Greg hesitated. "I need you to pull extra hours. Late nights, maybe some weekends."

David's stomach tightened.

A few months ago, he would have said yes without hesitation. He would have dropped everything—his workouts, his meal prep, his new routine—to prove himself at work.

But *that* version of him didn't exist anymore.

David exhaled. "I can put in extra effort. But my mornings? Those don't change."

Greg raised an eyebrow. "Carter, this is important."

David nodded. "I know. And I'll give it everything I've got—*after* my workout. That hour is *non-negotiable*."

Greg sighed, shaking his head. "You're serious?"

David met his gaze. "Yeah. Because I've learned that when I take care of myself first, I perform better. If you want my *best* work, then I need to keep the habits that make me *my best*."

Greg studied him for a moment, then—surprisingly—nodded.

"Alright. Do what you need to do. Just make sure we don't lose this account."

David stood, shaking his hand. "You've got my word."

As he left the conference room, he exhaled.

This was the real test.

Not just saying he had changed.

Living it.

And today?

He proved that his standards were *set in stone.*

Balance Without Compromise

The pressure was on.

The client was demanding, the project was behind schedule, and David's workload had doubled overnight.

But for the first time in his life, he wasn't letting *stress* dictate his decisions.

He wasn't skipping workouts. He wasn't eating like garbage just because it was "convenient." And he wasn't using long hours as an excuse to fall back into old habits.

Instead, he adapted.

Each morning, he hit the gym as planned.

He lifted heavier. Moved faster. Pushed harder.

And it showed.

Not just in his strength, but in his focus.

By the time he sat down at his desk, his mind was sharp, his energy steady.

While his coworkers dragged themselves through the day on caffeine and stress, he was *clear-headed.*

Mike noticed first.

"You're seriously not losing it over this deadline?" he asked one afternoon, slumping into the chair beside David's desk.

David smirked. "Nope."

Mike shook his head. "Man, I don't get it. Everyone else is cracking under pressure. You? You're just *good.*"

David leaned back. "Because I'm not letting work *own* me."

Mike frowned. "What does that mean?"

David exhaled. "It means I control *how* I show up. I start my day *my way.* No skipping workouts, no skipping meals, no sacrificing my health for a deadline."

Mike studied him. "And that actually helps?"

David grinned. "It doesn't just help—it changes *everything.*"

Mike sighed, rubbing his face. "Man, I need to start thinking like that."

David clapped him on the back. "Then stop thinking about it and *start doing it.*"

Mike chuckled. "Alright, alright. No more half-assing life."

David smirked. "Now you're getting it."

Because this wasn't about balance.

It was about *commitment.* And he wasn't compromising anymore.

MARK FLORY

The Real Strength Test

The long hours, the client demands, the endless revisions—it all built up like weights stacked on a bar.

David could handle it.

Because he had *trained* for this—not just in the gym, but in his *mind*.

But then, life threw another punch.

It was late when he got home. The house was quiet, except for the soft hum of the TV in the living room.

Lisa was curled up on the couch, scrolling through her phone.

She looked up as he walked in. "You're late."

David sighed, setting his bag down. "Yeah. Work's been crazy."

Lisa studied him for a moment. "And how long is that gonna be your excuse?"

David frowned. "What?"

Lisa sat up, crossing her arms. "Look, I get it. You're in a high-pressure situation. You're handling it better than ever. But lately? You've been here *less*. And when you are? Your mind is somewhere else."

David exhaled. "I'm just trying to make sure we don't lose this client, Lis."

Lisa nodded. "I know. And I love that you care about your work. But I also need to know you *care* about *us* just as much."

David swallowed hard.

He had been so focused on staying disciplined—on proving he could handle everything—that he hadn't stopped to *check in*.

Lisa sighed, her voice softer. "I'm proud of you, David. But don't let this new version of you *forget* what really matters."

David sat down beside her, rubbing his face.

She was right.

It wasn't just about work. It wasn't just about the gym.

It was about *the life he was building*.

He looked at Lisa, reaching for her hand. "You're right. I don't want to be the guy who only shows up at work or in the gym. I want to show up *here* too."

Lisa squeezed his fingers. "Then do that."

David exhaled.

Another challenge.

Another adjustment.

But if he had learned *anything*—it was that real strength wasn't just about lifting weights.

It was about *knowing where to put your energy.*

And tonight?

His energy was *here.*

Showing Up Where It Matters

The next morning, David did something different.

Instead of heading straight to the gym, he made coffee and sat with Lisa at the kitchen table.

She raised an eyebrow. "No workout first thing?"

David smirked, sipping his coffee. "I've got time."

Lisa leaned back. "Huh. You, the guy who has *zero* flexibility in his schedule, actually *adjusted?*"

David chuckled. "I realized something last night."

Lisa tilted her head. "Oh?"

David exhaled, setting his cup down. "Being disciplined isn't just about *what* I do—it's about *why* I do it. I'm building a better life, not just a stronger body."

Lisa smiled. "And part of that life includes more than just workouts and work?"

David nodded. "Yeah. It includes *this*. Us."

Lisa reached for his hand. "I love that."

David smirked. "Don't get used to me skipping the gym, though. I'm still going after this."

Lisa laughed. "I wouldn't expect anything less."

At work, things were chaotic.

But David was steady.

He didn't let stress derail him. Didn't let pressure dictate his actions.

And when Greg checked in on him that afternoon, he gave him the news.

"The client's happy," Greg said, leaning against the doorway. "You pulled it off."

David nodded. "Told you I would."

Greg smirked. "I gotta admit... I was worried you'd burn out."

David leaned back in his chair. "That's the old me. The guy who let stress run his life. Not anymore."

Greg studied him. "You really have changed."

David nodded. "Yeah. And I'm not going back."

Because this wasn't just about discipline.

It was about *living fully*—strong, focused, and *balanced*.

HEALING ME NOW

And now?
He had finally figured out how to do it.

CHAPTER
14

THE LIFESTYLE SHIFT

The Moment It Became Normal

David walked into the gym, but today, something felt different.
Not the weights. Not the routine. Not even the discipline.
It was *him*.
This wasn't a struggle anymore.
It wasn't a battle to stay motivated, to fight cravings, to force himself through workouts.
It was just *who he was now*.
Jake spotted him from across the room and smirked. "Damn, Carter. You're early."

David chuckled, setting his bag down. "Yeah, well, I got tired of waiting for you to catch up."

Jake laughed. "Look at you. Mr. Consistency."

David shrugged. "Honestly? I don't even think about it anymore. This is just my *life* now."

Jake nodded, grabbing a pair of weights. "That's the shift, man. When it's not about *trying*—it's just about *being*."

David exhaled. "Yeah... I feel that."

As he moved through his sets, he thought about how much had changed.

Not just his body.

His *mind*.

The way he handled stress. The way he structured his day. The way he made choices—not out of impulse, but out of *intention*.

Everything was *better*.

And for the first time in his life, he didn't feel like he was *chasing* health.

He was *living* it.

Jake tossed him a towel after the last set. "So, what's next?"

David smirked. "Same thing as always."

Jake raised an eyebrow. "Which is?"

David grinned.

"We keep going."

Because this wasn't just a fitness phase.

This was *forever*.

MARK FLORY

The Proof in the Mirror

Later that evening, David stood in front of the bathroom mirror, towel draped around his neck.

He had seen his reflection every day, but tonight—tonight, he really *looked.*

The man staring back at him wasn't the same guy from months ago.

His face was leaner. His shoulders were broader. His posture was stronger.

But beyond the physical changes, there was something else.

A presence. A confidence.

Not the kind that came from lifting weights, but from *knowing*—deep in his bones—that he had built this version of himself.

No shortcuts.
No gimmicks.
Just consistent, intentional work.

Lisa appeared in the doorway, watching him. "Checking yourself out again?"

David chuckled. "Just taking a second to appreciate it."

Lisa smiled, stepping forward. "You should."

David met her eyes in the mirror. "You ever worry I wouldn't stick with it?"

Lisa tilted her head. "Honestly? At first, yeah."

David nodded. "Me too."

Lisa wrapped her arms around him from behind. "But now? I don't worry at all. This is just *who you are.*"

David exhaled, resting a hand over hers. "Yeah... and I'm never going back."

Lisa squeezed him gently. "Good. Because I *love* this version of you."

David smirked. "Me too."

Because this wasn't about looking different.

It was about *being* different.

And for the first time in his life, he knew—

This was permanent.

The Unexpected Validation

The next day at work, David was in the middle of reviewing a report when Mike strolled over, a protein shake in hand.

"Alright, Carter," Mike said, leaning against the desk. "I gotta ask you something."

David smirked. "I feel like I should be worried."

Mike chuckled. "Nah, man. I just... I was talking to Sarah from accounting, and she said something that got me thinking."

David raised an eyebrow. "Oh?"

Mike took a sip of his shake. "She told me I *carry myself* differently now. Said I seem more focused. More *together*."

David grinned. "And?"

Mike exhaled. "And I realized something. I used to *wait* for motivation to hit before I made changes. But now? I just *do the work*."

David leaned back in his chair. "So, you're saying you get it now?"

Mike nodded. "Yeah, man. I *do*."

David smirked. "Took you long enough."

Mike laughed. "Shut up."

Then he got serious. "But for real... I wouldn't have gotten here without you pushing me."

David shook his head. "Nah. I didn't *push* you. I just set the standard. You chose to step up."

Mike nodded slowly. "Yeah. And now? I'm *never* stepping back down."

David smiled. "Good."

Because this wasn't just *his* transformation anymore.

It was a *ripple effect*.

And that?

That was bigger than any personal win.

The Final Piece of the Puzzle

That evening, David and Lisa went out for dinner—a rare night out, just the two of them.

They chose a quiet restaurant, the kind with warm lighting and soft music playing in the background.

Lisa studied the menu, glancing up at David with a smirk. "So, are you actually gonna let yourself enjoy this, or are you still in *full discipline* mode?"

David chuckled, setting his menu down. "I'm not on a 'diet,' Lis. I just make good choices."

Lisa smiled. "That's different from how you used to think about food."

David nodded. "Yeah... because I used to look at it like punishment. Like I had to suffer to get results." He leaned forward. "But now? I know it's not about extremes. It's about *balance*."

Lisa reached for his hand. "I love seeing you like this."

David tilted his head. "Like what?"

Lisa squeezed his fingers. "At peace with yourself."

David exhaled.

She was right.

For the first time in his life, he wasn't chasing some *temporary* version of himself.

This was *his life now*.

Not because he was forcing it.

Because he *chose* it.

The waiter arrived, and David grinned as he ordered a steak with roasted vegetables. A meal he *wanted*, not one dictated by guilt or obsession.

Because this wasn't about restriction.

It was about *freedom*.

And he had never felt lighter.

A Life Fully Lived

After dinner, David and Lisa took a slow walk through the city streets, the air cool, the hum of distant conversations filling the night.

Lisa glanced up at him. "So... what's next?"

David smirked. "What do you mean?"

Lisa shrugged. "You've built the habits. You've made the shift. But where do you *go* from here?"

David exhaled, stuffing his hands in his pockets. "Honestly? I just keep showing up. No end date, no finish line. Just *living* this way, because I love it."

Lisa smiled. "That's what makes this different, huh?"

David nodded. "Yeah. It's not about hitting a goal and stopping. It's about who I *am* now."

They stopped at a crosswalk, waiting for the light to change.

Lisa studied him. "I always believed in you, you know."

David smirked. "Even when I was the guy who hit snooze three times and lived off takeout?"

Lisa chuckled. "Even then."

David shook his head. "Well, I'm never going back to that guy."

Lisa squeezed his arm. "I know."

The light changed, and they crossed the street together.

David felt the steady strength in his body, the clarity in his mind, the *purpose* in his steps.

This wasn't just a *transformation*.

It was his *life*.

And every day, he was choosing to live it fully.

CHAPTER 15

THE HEALTHY MINDSET

The Power of Choice

David sat on the back patio, a cup of coffee in hand, watching the sunrise.

It had been months since he started this journey.

And yet, it still felt like it was just *beginning*.

Not because he was struggling.

Not because he was trying to *maintain* something.

But because he had built a life he *wanted* to keep living.

Lisa stepped outside, wrapping herself in a sweater. "You're up early."

David smirked. "Habit."

She sat beside him, tucking her legs under her. "You ever stop and think about how far you've come?"

David took a sip of coffee, nodding. "Yeah. And you know what I realized?"

Lisa tilted her head. "What?"

David exhaled. "It all came down to *one thing*."

Lisa raised an eyebrow. "Discipline?"

David shook his head. "Choice."

Lisa smiled. "Go on."

David leaned back in his chair. "Every day, I get to *choose* how I show up. Choose what I eat. Choose whether I move my body. Choose how I handle stress. It's all just choices stacked on top of each other."

Lisa nodded. "And now those choices feel *normal*?"

David smirked. "Yeah. Because I stopped negotiating with myself. Stopped waiting to 'feel' like doing the right thing. I just *do it*."

Lisa reached for his hand. "That's why this time was different."

David exhaled. "Yeah. And that's why I *know* I'll never go back."

Because healing—real, lasting healing—wasn't about a quick fix.

It was about waking up *every day* and making the choice to keep moving forward.

And now?

That choice was *easy*.

The Strength in Simplicity

David finished his coffee, letting the warmth settle inside him.

It wasn't just about the drink. It was about *the moment*—this quiet space where he could reflect, appreciate, and *be present*.

Lisa watched him, a soft smile playing on her lips. "You seem different."

David smirked. "Well, I *am* different."

She shook her head. "No, I mean... you're at peace."

David exhaled, nodding. "Yeah. Because I finally get it."

Lisa leaned in. "Get what?"

David set his mug down. "That healing, growth, *change*—it's all simple. Not easy, but *simple*."

Lisa tilted her head. "Explain."

David stretched his arms, feeling the steady strength in his body. "It's not about chasing some perfect version of myself. It's about showing up. Making the next right decision. Sticking to the basics."

Lisa smirked. "So all of this—months of effort—just came down to *simplicity*?"

David nodded. "Yeah. No shortcuts, no hacks. Just consistent, simple actions, repeated over time."

Lisa chuckled. "I think people spend their whole lives looking for a magic answer. And here you are, saying it's just *showing up*?"

David grinned. "Exactly. The hard part isn't knowing *what* to do—it's *doing it* every day, even when it's boring."

Lisa exhaled, watching the morning sky shift from dark blue to soft gold. "I like this version of you."

David reached for her hand. "Me too."

Because healing wasn't about finding a secret formula.

It was about *choosing*—every single day—to live better.

And that?

That was the simplest truth of all.

Becoming an Example

Later that afternoon, David headed to the gym, but this time, something was different.

Mike was already there, warming up—something that never used to happen.

David smirked, crossing his arms. "Look at you, showing up *early*."

Mike chuckled, rolling his shoulders. "Gotta keep up with you, man."

David nodded toward the weights. "So, what's the plan today?"

Mike grabbed a kettlebell. "Same as always. Keep pushing forward."

David smiled. That was the answer he had been waiting for.

Because Mike wasn't just *trying* anymore.

He *was* this now.

And it hit David—his journey wasn't just about himself anymore.

People were watching.

People were learning.

He had become an example—not because he had set out to be, but because he had *lived* the truth.

Mike picked up the kettlebell and smirked. "Come on, Carter. No slacking today."

David chuckled. "I wouldn't dream of it."

They started their workout, side by side.

And as the weights moved, the sweat dripped, and the muscles burned, David realized something.

This wasn't about *finishing* a journey.

It was about *living* it.

Every day.

Every choice.

Because the real impact wasn't just in what he had achieved.

It was in *who he was helping become better along the way.*

The Legacy of Discipline

As David and Mike finished their last set, the gym's steady hum of clanking weights and low music filled the air.

Mike dropped onto a bench, shaking his head. "Man... remember when this used to feel impossible?"

David smirked, tossing him a towel. "Yeah. And now it's just *normal*."

Mike wiped the sweat from his face. "You ever think about what would've happened if you never started?"

David exhaled. "All the time."

He thought about the old version of himself—the guy who hit snooze, who made excuses, who *let life happen* instead of *owning it.*

That guy was gone.

And it wasn't because of some overnight change.

It was because of the daily *discipline*—the choice to show up, no matter what.

Mike stretched his arms. "So what now? We just... keep doing this forever?"

David grinned. "Pretty much."

Mike chuckled. "You're okay with that?"

David nodded. "Yeah. Because discipline isn't a *punishment.* It's *freedom.*"

Mike raised an eyebrow. "Freedom?"

David leaned forward, elbows on his knees. "Yeah. Freedom from feeling tired all the time. Freedom from doubting myself. Freedom from wondering if I'll ever be the guy I want to be."

Mike sat with that for a moment. Then he nodded. "Damn. Never thought about it like that."

David clapped him on the back. "That's why you stick with it. Because you don't just get stronger—you get *better.*"

Mike stood up, cracking his neck. "Alright then. Guess we keep going."

David grinned. "You *know* it."

Because this wasn't a phase.

It was a *lifestyle.*

And now, there was no turning back.

HEALING ME NOW

The Journey Never Ends

That evening, David sat on the back patio, watching the sunset paint the sky in shades of orange and gold.

Lisa stepped outside, handing him a cup of tea. "Long day?"

David smiled, taking the cup. "A good one."

She sat beside him, tucking her legs under her. "You look... different."

David smirked. "Again?"

Lisa chuckled. "Yeah. But not because of the gym. Not even because of the discipline."

She met his gaze. "You're *settled*. Like you're exactly where you're supposed to be."

David took a slow sip of tea, letting her words sink in.

Because she was right.

For years, he had chased the *idea* of a better version of himself.

But now?

Now, he wasn't *chasing* anymore.

He was *living it.*

No quick fixes. No end goals.

Just showing up. Every day.

For his health. For his mindset. For his future.

Lisa leaned her head on his shoulder. "So... what's next?"

David exhaled, smiling. "Tomorrow. The same as today. And the next day. And the next."

Lisa smirked. "That simple?"

David nodded. "Yeah. Because the journey never ends."

She squeezed his hand. "I love that."

David looked out at the sky, feeling the quiet certainty settle deep inside him.

Because this wasn't just about *healing*.

It was about *living*—fully, completely, with purpose.

And for the first time, he knew—

He had finally become the man he was always meant to be.

FINAL THOUGHTS

Your Journey to Healing Never Ends

I f there's one thing I want you to take away from this book, it's this: **healing is not a destination—it's a lifelong journey.** It's not about achieving some final form of peak health and never struggling again. It's about showing up for yourself every day, making small, meaningful changes, and embracing the process of transformation.

There will be days when you feel on top of the world—when your energy is high, your mind is clear, and your body moves with strength and purpose. And there will be days when it feels like nothing is changing, when old habits try to creep back in, and when doubt whispers in your ear. Those are the moments that define your journey. **Those are the moments where you must choose persistence over perfection.**

There Is No One-Size-Fits-All Approach

One of the biggest lies in the health industry is that there is only **one right way** to achieve your goals. That's simply not true. What works for one person may not work for another. Some people thrive on the **Keto diet**, while others feel their best following the **DASH diet**. Some gain strength through **heavy lifting**, while others build resilience using **resistance bands** or **bodyweight exercises**. Some sleep best with guided meditation, while others find relief through breathwork or changing their nighttime routine.

The key to success isn't blindly following someone else's blueprint—it's about **discovering what works for you**. That's why the **4 Pillars of Healing** exist:

1. **Nutrition** – Experiment, track what fuels your body best, and adjust accordingly.
2. **Physical Activity** – Move in a way that strengthens you, whether it's weight training, yoga, or simply walking.
3. **Sleep** – Prioritize rest and recovery; your body does its deepest healing while you sleep.
4. **Self-Improvement** – Your mindset is your most powerful tool. Develop habits that support growth and long-term success.

Start Where You Are

So where do you begin? Right where you are. You don't need to overhaul your entire life overnight. You don't have to run miles to get in shape. **Start by walking.** Walking is one of the most powerful tools you have—it's free, it's easy on the body, and it benefits both your physical and mental health. A simple 15-minute walk can clear your mind, reduce stress, and get your body moving. And when you're ready, you can build from there.

Small steps lead to big changes. Add one healthy meal to your day. Go to bed 30 minutes earlier. Swap out one negative thought for a positive affirmation. **These small actions, repeated consistently, will change your life.**

My Journey Continues, Too

I won't pretend I have it all figured out. **I'm still learning, still growing, and still healing every day.** My body is getting stronger, my mind is getting clearer, and I'm feeling better than I have in years. But I still have pain sometimes. There are still days when I struggle. The difference now is that those days are fewer and farther between. And when they do come, I know I have the tools to keep moving forward.

You have those tools now, too. You have the knowledge, the mindset, and the foundation to create lasting change. The question is—**will you take action?**

You Are Not Alone

The path to healing is not meant to be walked alone. **You are part of a community of people who are on this journey with you.** At HealingMeNow.com, you'll find resources, insights, and encouragement to keep you moving forward. More importantly, you'll find **a community that understands your struggles, celebrates your wins, and supports you through the tough days.**

Your journey doesn't end here—it's just beginning. And the best part? **You get to decide what happens next.**

So take a step. Keep moving forward. Trust yourself. Because every small action you take today is a step toward the stronger, healthier, and more purpose-filled life you deserve.

This is your journey. This is your time. And you are ready.

Let's keep healing, together.

Mark Flory – Author & Holistic Health Advocate

Mark is a former professional athlete turned holistic health advocate, and has a degree specializing in **Mind-Body Transformational Psychology**. After years of battling chronic pain from his sports career, he discovered the power of **nutrition, movement, and mindset** in healing the body. Now pursuing a **secondary degree in Nutritional Health**, Mark is dedicated to helping others over 40 reduce inflammation, regain energy, and achieve lasting wellness.

For more, visit [**www.healingmenow.com**].

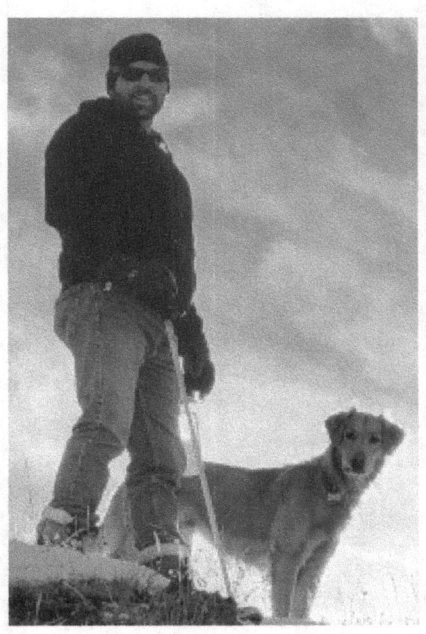

www.ingramcontent.com/pod-product-compliance
Lightning Source LLC
Chambersburg PA
CBHW010330030426
42337CB00026B/4885